A
CAREGIVER'S
JOURNEY

SELF-CARE FOR CAREGIVERS OF LOVED ONES
WITH DEMENTIA AND ALZHEIMER'S

A CAREGIVER'S JOURNEY

SELF-CARE FOR CAREGIVERS OF LOVED ONES WITH DEMENTIA AND ALZHEIMER'S

FROM A LOVING SON'S PERSPECTIVE
ERIC JAMES MILLER

CASTLE HORSE PRESS

ISBN: 978-0-9897363-1-2

First Edition, April 2021
Printed in the United States

CASTLE HORSE PRESS
Las Vegas, Nevada

www.thecaregivingproject.com

TO

SYLVIA ROSE MILLER,
MY MOTHER,
MY BEST FRIEND AND
MY GREATEST TEACHER

*"Fasten your seatbelts,
it's going to be a bumpy ride"*

– ATTRIBUTED TO BETTE DAVIS – *ALL ABOUT EVE* (1950)

CONTENTS

INTRODUCTION

This book is for those who find themselves in a primary or secondary caregiver role for anyone suffering from Alzheimer's or other types of dementia.

Caring for someone suffering from dementia is incredibly challenging. Whether it's the mean-spirited, toxic kind, or the sweet, forgetful old lady/old man kind associated with Alzheimer's, or, as in my mother's case, a combination of both, the sliding scale of good days can quickly take over a caregiver's life.

I wasn't prepared for it. But I wrote this book to help others prepare for it.

I hope this book will serve as the roadmap I wish I had. I hope it will help caregivers of dementia and Alzheimer's patients know what to expect. From the things they are likely to hear, to the difficult decisions they will likely face, to knowing how to plan for the future. Most of all, I want other caregivers to remember the importance of caring for themselves on their own caregiving journeys. Because I almost didn't.

EJM
Las Vegas, Nevada
August 2020

CHAPTER 1

MY MOTHER'S TIMELINE

My mother was an amazing woman. She was born on a 300-acre farm in western Pennsylvania in 1923 and had a full and vibrant, some might even say groundbreaking life up until she started being consumed at age 94 by what her doctors diagnosed as Alzheimer's Disease. But before the forgetfulness and debilitating physical decay of Alzheimer's set in, for ten-plus years she, and I as her primary caregiver and legal guardian, were challenged with her increasingly toxic episodes of dementia.

By describing the timeline of her life, I hope to both honor my mother and provide some perspective on how the neurological decay she suffered from fundamentally changed her as a person. Understanding her timeline will also provide context and the ability to relate certain events to the many challenges that I faced and the discoveries that I made as a caregiver for someone suffering Alzheimer's/dementia.

For most of her life my mother was loved (or at least very well-liked) and respected by just about everyone, she met and she did more with her high school education than most people do with their master's degrees.

Her first job was working at a munitions factory in Latrobe, Pennsylvania during World War II. After the war was over and all four of her brothers who went overseas came back as heroes, she was hired by the Arthur Murray Dance Company to go on the road and be a showcase dancer for new studios they were opening. She ended up in St. Louis, enrolled in airline school and after flying with TWA a bit, she decided living out of her suitcase wasn't for her so she applied for and got transferred to air traffic control in Washington, D.C.

Smart, young, and popular in a big city bustling with exciting things to do and new opportunities in the early 1950's, she felt "fenced in" by the stressful demands of working in air traffic control so enrolled in secretarial school. After a stint in the secretarial pool of the FBI, she landed an even better paying job at the National Association of Home Builders.

She met my father at a trade show, got married and led a busy, fun, urban life in a growing, vibrant city, while staying connected to her large family (7 brothers and 3 sisters) scattered in western Pennsylvania and New York. Since she had been told by doctors from an early age that she would never be able to have children, she focused on her career. She got lured away from the NAHB and became a legal secretary for prominent D.C. attorney Bernard "Bernie" Margolius. Then, a year or so after the surprise birth of me, she was lured away from the Margolius firm to another very prominent D.C. law firm, Wilmer, Cutler & Pickering.

After divorcing my father for reasons I'd rather not go into here, my mother found herself a single mom in her forties with sole custody of a young boy during the increasingly tumultuous Sixties. She was faced with some very tough decisions. She couldn't keep working the 60-80 hour work weeks demanded of a top legal secretary and raise me by herself at the same time. So she retreated back to her small hometown in Pennsylvania into countless open arms, but limited rural opportunities.

Rural life was not for my mother after her jet set years in St. Louis and Washington, D.C.. The siren call of big city life beckoned her to return. But it had to be on new terms because of me. She was wanted back at her old job at Wilmer, Cutler & Pickering, and at Margolius's firm, but she couldn't commit to the long hours because of me.

Instead, she used her legal experience and glowing recommendations from her former employers to land a low paying job with set hours with the Montgomery County government. She found a small, ground floor, one-bedroom apartment to rent on Lee Avenue in Takoma Park, Maryland for us that she could afford on the modest salary, came back to Pennsylvania to get me (I had been staying with her sister and husband, my awesome Aunt Bessie and Uncle Ray, while she looked for work) and she moved us back to the D.C. area (for which I will be eternally, eternally grateful).

The top bunk of a sturdy bunk bed, probably bought on store credit, was waiting for me when we got there, along with a few other pieces of start-all-over-again furniture. About a year after we moved in, she traded in the old blue Studebaker (I think it was a '58) that I loved but can barely remember and took out a small loan for a shiny, gently used, white 1962 Ford Falcon with a glossy red vinyl interior.

I'm sure it wasn't easy making ends meet. But I never, ever realized what she accomplished on her $150/week salary until I started making my own money years later.

Fortunately, she had a large, loving, and supportive family just four hours away that we visited often. Plus, our little 3-story, 6-unit red brick building was tucked into the downward slope of a hill next to another little 3-story, 6-unit red brick building next door. The wife of a friendly couple who lived there became my first, non-family member babysitter and Vicki, their daughter, who was two years older than me but only one year ahead of me in school, became my new schoolmate.

The Cunninghams were great. We went everywhere as a pack of five together. Movie nights, pizza nights, picnics, day trips to the Potomac, the monuments downtown, the Chesapeake Bay and even all the way and back to Ocean City on the Atlantic shore sometimes. But then our little neighborhood of towering and not so towering apartment buildings started to change from cozy, friendly, and safe to not so safe. John, Jeannie, and Vicki moved to Virginia to be closer to the carpet store he owned in Fairfax. Uncertainty returned I'm sure, but again, I never knew it. Money was still tight. No doubt because for the first time in my mother's life she was in a workplace where promotions were <u>not</u> always based on merit.

She felt "trapped" working for the county government. I remember overhearing that word when we would visit Pennsylvania for family reunions and major holiday picnics. But instead of wallowing in the fact that the dynamics and opportunities there weren't likely to improve, she took on the task of looking for something better. Her best friend at the time, Anna Belle, a friend she had made back when she was a legal secretary in the Margolius law firm, talked to her boss and he said my mother could get a job back at the firm whenever she wanted because they were growing in new directions and they "needed" her.

But even though I was seven and looking out for myself more and more by then, my mother knew that long hours were inevitable and would quickly create a new set of problems for her. So, instead of taking a good job that paid well but demanded long hours, she became the neighborhood Avon woman at night, after dinner, to make extra money.

She hated it, but with her usual grit and common sense, she killed it.

Mrs. Murphy, a kindly old grandmother who lived upstairs with her divorced daughter and granddaughter looked after me after school for whatever my mother could afford to pay her and I stayed in and did my homework on the two or three nights a week my mother made her Avon rounds. My mother and the grandmother's daughter, although in similar situations as single mothers, did NOT get along. Shirley was probably almost fifteen years younger than my mother and acted like they were in direct competition with each other. Over what, I have no idea. Looking back, I can see that Shirely probably felt intimidated and no doubt a little, or a lot, envious.

It didn't help that my mother had a sharp tongue for anyone who "didn't use the brains God gave a duck."

Because of her success, Avon wanted to expand her territory. They offered to give her a better territory in a more affluent neighborhood and hire a new rep to work under her that she could train and manage to cover her current territory. But door-to-door sales didn't appeal to my mother. On top of that, although she never talked about it, it couldn't have been safe. It was largely a cash business and petty crime was on the rise in Takoma Park at that time. She had to have known she was a target.

The Falcon got traded in for a brand new, lemon yellow 1967 Dodge Dart sometime in 1968. She had purposely waited until the new model year cars came out to get a good deal on a prior year model. In 1969, Bernie Margolius, my mother's old boss, recommended her to one of his new business partners, Melvin Lenkin, a commercial builder in D.C. who was looking for someone with organizational, legal, and accounting savvy. No doubt the account management success she had with Avon played into getting her new job with the Lenkin Company. It paid so much better than the one she had with the county, she was able to quit doing the Avon gig.

That summer my mother "splurged" again and bought us our first television set because she felt it was important for me to see the first man to walk on the moon. It was a 15" portable B&W Zenith with two long, retractable "rabbit ears" that looked like Ray Walston's antennae on a show I was about to fall in love with called

"My Favorite Martian" that starred him and Bill Bixby. I remember she brought the set home the day before Apollo 11 landed, set it next to the radio on the credenza in our modest living room in front of the blue, pull-out bed couch, and I absolutely couldn't believe it.

We had caught up to the future. We were living in the future.

She called it witnessing history. I repeated what I had heard in school and called it looking into the future. She smiled and gave me a long, smothering hug as we stood in front of that little TV set and she told me "the future starts from now."

The Apollo 11 mission was of course a big deal in my elementary school. No doubt partly due to the fact that it was a very big deal for the U.S. government and we lived literally less than a mile from the Maryland/D.C. border. We were certainly by no means the only ones on our block with a TV. A lot of people had TVs, even color TVs (!!) but it felt to me like we were part of Mission Control to be able to watch Neil Armstrong descend that ladder and say his immortal words, "One small step for man, one giant leap for mankind."

Less than a year later, the Lenkin company moved offices and we made a giant leap of our own from our tiny, one-bedroom apartment in Takoma Park to a giant, top floor, two-bedroom one on Battery Lane in upscale Bethesda, Maryland. My mother could walk to work and the bus that took me to my new school stopped right down the street.

By this point you can probably tell that my mother was a smart, independent, force of sheer will and determination.

What I probably haven't made clear is that she was funny and generous with a quick tongue for some people and an even quicker tongue for others.

I loved her very much.

And so did most people who met her.

For the next twenty-three years she lived happily and joyfully in the beautiful, L-shaped apartment on the top floor that had a big, sweeping view of the western sky out the living room and dining room windows. Over the years she decorated it lavishly to her taste, with a mirrored wall and crystal chandelier in the dining room, a seven-foot lemon yellow velvet couch, white shag carpeting, a six-piece matching Early American furniture set for my room and an eight-piece, light blue, Queen Anne furniture set for hers. She bought a complete set of gold-embossed Lennox china, and with my lucrative apartment-building paper routes for *The Washington Star* and *The Washington Post* (which she helped me with on weekends) I added to her beautiful collection of Waterford crystal that was used for frequent special occasions. She became the accounting and office manager at the Lenkin Company with a staff of four reporting to her and when I got my learner's permit when I was 15, I inherited the Dart and she bought a brand new, forest green Chevy Malibu that quickly got traded in for a beautiful, two-tone, 1983 Oldsmobile Cutlass Brougham with plush teal interior.

For a hobby and for exercise she enrolled in evening ballroom dance classes and it wasn't long before she was competing in and winning competitions in her age group. A few years after I graduated from college, she retired from the Lenkin Company and took her sister, my Aunt Bessie, to Sweden to visit the hometown where their mother had been born. Not long after returning from what turned out to be the first of many trips she took (by herself mostly) to Sweden, she saw an ad in the paper for ushers at the Kennedy Center. Being a lifelong fan of dance and music and theater, she made her new part-time gig a central part of her life along with her ballroom dancing and frequent trips to Pennsylvania, New York, and Florida to visit family.

In 1993, at age seventy, after visiting me twice in L.A. and falling in love with the warm climate and close proximity to the beautiful and majestic Pacific Ocean, I helped her pack up her life in Bethesda and move into a nice, conveniently located apartment in Eagle Rock. It was close to where I lived in Los Feliz, and to the museums and picturesque downtown area of Pasadena which I had already introduced her to during one of her previous visits.

Less than a year after she got settled in, the Northridge Earthquake struck. Although Eagle Rock was about 25 miles from the epicenter of the giant 6.7 quake, it was in a direct line along the same ridge of mountains so she felt the earthquake (and quick succession of large aftershocks) far more than I did in Venice Beach where I had moved to by then.

While most of her expensive Lennox china and Waterford crystal was falling out of her china cabinet and crashing to the floor upon itself in a cacophonous crescendo I can only imagine, I was sitting up in my bed looking out the window, amazed that I was able to see the pavement of Electric Avenue buckling up and down like an out of control conveyor belt flying off its hinges.

She certainly had every right to cry that morning and for weeks afterwards. Like so many other Californians at the time, natives and transplants, she did. It was probably the first time in her life she felt completely helpless and out of control, and it's possible that singularly traumatic event may have triggered the change that was to come in her personality.

When her lease was up, she moved into a new apartment in Burbank to get away from the apartment in Eagle Rock which she said constantly reminded her of the earthquake. It made sense to me. When I had called her after the quake to see if she felt it, she was crying hysterically. I rushed over and cleaned up the thousands of dollars of china and crystal and everything else that had been tossed around in her apartment, so I knew she had been through quite a traumatic experience.

While helping her pack her things to move, I discovered a tiny white notepad with columns of small numbers written on it on one of the end tables next to her couch. For months she had been obsessively watching the local news and writing down every minor aftershock they mentioned. After I got her moved and settled into Burbank, about six months after the quake, she had a minor heart attack while we were walking to lunch in Venice. A week after that a heart surgeon put a stint in her heart to strengthen some arterial damage. Not entirely pleased with her progress, a few months later, he put in another stint. A little more than a year after the quake struck, she had triple bypass surgery and I found several more notepads with pages and pages of neat columns of penciled numbers on the end table next to her couch ...

1.2

1.4

2.1

1.7

1.3

She didn't even bother to write down the date or the time of each little aftershock. Just its magnitude. I found out years later from talking with her doctors that major life events can often be triggers for the onset of Alzheimer's or other dementia. The stress associated with the event somehow triggers the onset of sticky platelets in the brain to start forming. More about those nasty little platelets in CHAPTER 3.

As I found out myself later,

Stress can kill.

Sometimes fast.

Sometimes slow.

It can strike on the most tense and challenging days.

Or, it can strike on the most serene and idyllic morning or afternoon.

Although my mother made a remarkable recovery from the triple bypass surgery for someone who was over 70 years old, for the next ten years she had an on again/off again, love/hate relationship towards southern California which in retrospect I find totally understandable.

The first time she moved back to the D.C. area was in the summer of 1996. Dorothy, one of her Kennedy Center friends, found her a nice, high rise apartment in Arlington, Virginia and I reluctantly helped my mother move back to the D.C. area. She was welcomed back as an usher at the Kennedy Center and quickly was back in her old, comfortable routine with her longtime friends Dorothy, Alan, Charlene and others. California wasn't for her. After what she had been through with the Northridge Earthquake and triple bypass it seemed totally understandable. They assured me they would look after her and they each absolutely kept their word.

I talked with her every week. But after just one winter, she pined for warm and sunny southern California and said that she had made a mistake trying to go back to a life that wasn't there anymore for her. I couldn't blame her. There was a vacancy in the Burbank apartment she had lived in before so once again I helped her move across the country. She settled in quickly, and through a local recreation center she discovered country-western line dancing and instantly fell in love with it. But the dread of "the next big one" compelled her back to the same apartment building in Arlington two years later because D.C. was her "home," not California.

She lasted two winters the second time — but was back in Burbank in 2001.

I jokingly started calling her a move-a-holic. Between 1993 and 2001 she moved back and forth across the country five times. Five times! I started to wonder if the threat of earthquakes and the cold and icy Mid-Atlantic winters were really the root causes of her inability to make a decision and stick to it.

Although that might sound like irrational behaviour, I think it was more a sense of feeling like she didn't have any purpose in life anymore. After living such an intense and driven life, I think the relative comfort she had in retirement was simply boring for her. I wouldn't say my mother started losing grip with reality until around the time she turned eighty (80) years young in 2003. Up until that point she was the proverbial little old lady from Pasadena (except that she lived between Burbank and Arlington!) driving everywhere in her classic, two-tone Oldsmobile Cutlass Supreme Brougham, going to museums, going out to eat with friends, entering (and winning!) competitive dance competitions, flying on her own from California to New York and Florida to visit relatives, entertaining, and generally being the life of every party. She lived on her own comfortably, managed her own modest finances, told funny stories about her past, herself and others. She was smart and interesting and fiercely independent just like she had always been, and just about everyone who met her fell in love with her.

No one could believe she was 80 years old. She walked, ran, and danced circles around people ten years younger. But then, she started dropping the f-bomb for the first time in her life and having random, extremely bitter, delusional meltdowns about once every other month. She started falling into woeful pits of despair that lasted four or five days and then were gone. She periodically lashed out at everyone around her. But most of the time she was still the person I had known for almost forty years.

When she started saying things like "I just want it to be over" and "I want to be with Pop again" (her father) I attributed it to a spiritual satisfaction with her life and her belief that she had been here before and would be again. But when she turned on all of her line dancing friends in Pasadena and Burbank and suddenly announced that she "hated" dancing, I knew something wasn't right. But I didn't know what, or how, to deal with it or even what to say. I was living with my soon-to-be wife Laura in Redondo Beach by then and she thought it would help if my mother lived closer to us, so she helped find my mother a cute, little one-bedroom apartment within walking distance of us.

The prospect of moving always cheered my mother up and it worked like a charm. But less than a week after she was all moved in, the despair, regret, and morbidity returned full force.

Her mental state was difficult to understand because aside from the increasingly frequent pits of despair and/or bitter rage that she fell into, my mother was still extremely competent, healthy and independent in every other area of her life. The L.A. traffic had become a bit daunting for her and after she had a minor traffic accident I made sure she got a good price for her beloved car, and she eagerly and happily learned all the ins and outs of the L.A. transit system. She loved it and it became pretty much her favorite topic of conversation for a while.

*Her first major break from reality
was jarring, sudden,
and completely unprovoked.*

Laura's parents came to California from Georgia to celebrate Christmas with us in 2004. They arrived a few days beforehand to enjoy some sights, and the five of us had a wonderful meal on Christmas Eve at one of our favorite restaurants in Redondo. My mother had met Laura's parents earlier that year and even stayed with them in their home in Georgia. They got along fantastically well and the Christmas Eve dinner had been nothing but thoroughly enjoyable. My mother had been a big part of the plans we had to cook Christmas Day dinner at our place, but right before I was to pick her up (as previously scheduled) she called and announced that she wasn't coming. She had a whole list of reasons, not one of which was grounded in reality. She accused me and Laura and Laura's parents of conspiring against her and laughing behind her back at her and "hating" her and being "embarrassed" to be around her. I tried to reason with her. I tried to remind her what a pleasant time she had had in Georgia and just the previous night but nothing worked. She was full of so much venom and quiet, simmering rage that I felt like I was in some sort of surreal Monty Python skit. Finally, I relented. I told her I wasn't going to make her "endure" anything that she didn't want to so I wished her a Merry Christmas, she said f-you (which was equally surreal because she had only just recently started dropping f-bombs after never, ever using them before in her life) and hung up.

I tried to explain to my future in-laws, and Laura tried to help by recounting the rollercoaster she had experienced with my mother moving her from Burbank to Redondo, but I'm sure it didn't seem as comical to them as it did to us. I blamed it on my mother's meds not working. Which probably made them wonder if my mother's psychosis was hereditary (the jury's still out on that lol).

My mother never apologized to me or to Laura or to Laura's parents. She did ask the following week when I called to see how she was doing (I thought it best to give her some space) if we had a "nice" dinner and if Laura's parents made it back to Georgia okay, but that was the end of it.

A week after that tepidly friendly phone call, she was pretty much her old self, talking about where she had been on the subway and what she had been cooking up in her kitchen. By the time Laura and I got married in November of 2005 all had been forgotten and my mother had a grand and glorious time celebrating in Las Vegas with us, her sister Alma who travelled from her home in New York, our friends, many of whom she already knew, and Laura's parents.

Then, two months after Laura and I got married, my mother announced on the steps of our beautiful Redondo Beach apartment overlooking Santa Monica Bay on a warm and sunny Saturday afternoon in early January 2006, while she was petting our golden retriever puppy Zazzy who she dearly, dearly loved, that she had made arrangements to move back to Arlington the following month.

I reminded her the last time she moved back that I had said it was the last time I would lift a finger to help her move across the country again. She didn't care. She accused us of not wanting her around anymore. She accused us of countless other crazy things and transgressions just like she had a little more than a year earlier at Christmas 2004. After arguing with her for an hour I finally gave up. Laura went inside and cried, trying to make sense of the situation while I just shook my head and said don't bother because there wasn't any sense in it to be found.

My mother had "decided" she was going to be her youngest sister Alma's "problem" now. Her "only true friends in this world," meaning her Kennedy Center friends, would take care of her. Which again, they promised me sincerely that they would do, even though each and every one of them had spent long, long hours on the telephone with her trying to talk her out of it because they knew that nothing she said was true and that I was doing an excellent job of seeing that she was safe and being looked after.

But nothing anyone said could reach her. So, at 82 years old, my mother sent a check for first and last month's rent to the same apartment building in Arlington that she had already moved in and out of twice, packed up everything in her apartment, hired movers, and moved back across the country for the third time completely by herself with no help from me or anyone else.

I'll let you guess who got a wilting and withering phone call of regret less than a week later.

Her meltdowns went from occurring every other month to occurring monthly, like clockwork, either right before or right after each calendar change. There was little I could do from almost 4,000 miles away except listen. She made it clear on numerous occasions that she didn't want my help or my advice and began lamenting more and more frequently that she just wanted "everything" to be over. I asked if she was still taking the anti-depressants her doctor had prescribed, and she said yes but that they weren't working. I suspected that she wasn't taking them anymore but had no way to be sure. She said she was going to go live with her sister Alma in Florida. I didn't like the idea of her living by herself anymore, so I agreed that sounded like a good idea to me even though I knew it wasn't.

The upside to my mother being gone (in more ways than one) was that Laura and I had the space to realize that we had grown weary of the L.A. rat race too. Although we both had good jobs, the hope of buying a home in a neighborhood that we liked seemed remote at best. We were looking at six-hundred-thousand dollar tear-downs thirty and forty miles from where we worked and not loving the idea at all. Then one night, after returning home from dinner, Laura suggested we look into moving to Las Vegas. We had gotten to know the city a little from having our wedding there and it seemed like a fun and growing city, on top of being much, much more affordable. Later that year we did. We moved into a gorgeous 3-bedroom home in the Green Valley Ranch area of Henderson, and we both parlayed our accounting experience and went to work for Robert Half.

My mother came to visit that Christmas, fell in love with the warm, dry climate and the chance to explore a new place, and after I found her a nice apartment in an active 55+ retirement community she packed up her things again, hired movers and moved back across the country all by herself again. This time at age 84.

She loved it. At first. But then her meltdowns and bursts of rage co-mingled with woeful despair started occurring about every two weeks. That every other week pattern lasted three more years until the meltdowns became weekly. By that point I began to dread the sound of my phone ringing. I also started dreading calling her and going over to see how she was doing because no matter what plans and activities we did together, no matter how much fun she had on one of the community bus excursions to the casinos or other sights to see, no matter how many penny slot jackpots she hit, it was never good enough to keep her happy for very long.

Her reasoning became increasingly paranoid. The woeful pits of despair became more frequent and even darker. We got her more mood-stabilizing medications but nothing seemed to work for very long. I checked the bottles to make sure she was taking them, but she was smart, not absent-minded. She easily could have been throwing the pills out rather than taking them just to fool me. Regardless of why it was happening, more and more she became increasingly toxic towards everyone around her until that was her primary personality trait.

The change accelerated slowly but steadily until ten years later, she still looked the same on the outside, but she was not the same person. By 2016 she had become a different person. A volatile person. A toxic person. A person most people could only stand to be around on a limited basis.

She severed every single friendship she had ever had. Everyone in Arlington and Washington had "betrayed" her. She poisoned ties with her family, although fortunately her sister Alma was becoming forgetful too, so that worked in my mother's favor when she found she had no one else to complain to. Every new person that she met was usually greeted with disdain or outright derision. Eventually, the person who had been my mother was utterly and completely gone. Even when she was standing right in front of me.

Long before she wasn't able to live on her own anymore, long before she wasn't able to balance her checkbook, or cook for herself, or walk unassisted — some of the early signs of Alzheimer's disease — she exhibited other traits commonly (and historically) referred to as dementia.

Toxic behaviours and mean-as-piss character traits that got people institutionalized fifty ago. But today, thanks to medical advancements and tech for living advancements that make day-to-day living easier than ever for everyone, people are living much longer, healthier lives than they were a hundred years ago. As a society, we have learned how to not only slow, but improve, the physical deterioration associated with the aging process. But as a society, we are just beginning to understand the science and implications of the mental aspects of aging.

My mother's dementia started long before the early symptoms of Alzheimer's began to manifest. She didn't just have Alzheimer's disease. Her slide into the frail, forgetful, confused and disoriented aspects commonly associated with the disease took fifteen (15!) long, torturous years.

I watched my mother become someone I no longer knew.

Her experience, or mine as her caregiver for that matter, was not unique. Millions of older adults are living with some form of dementia. Because people are living longer lives than ever before, as a society we are increasingly monetizing the nuances of aging. Instead of cramming older people into depressing nursing homes where they are heavily sedated and hooked to feeding tubes as my grandmother was for the last ten years of her life, we're trying to value and find ways to restore dignity to older adults. Instead of being half-forgotten, or visited by only a handful of duty-bound relatives whenever it's least inconvenient, older adults today are more often living in cheery, assisted-living communities where they have a good quality of life and can interact with their families and each other rather than just being stored in a room waiting to die.

As an older adult human who is experiencing some early signs of aging myself, (I make more noises getting in and out of my car these days) I would argue that new attitudes about quality of life for older adults is a good thing. However, the collective benefit of prolonging all of our lives directly impacts our individual lives when our parents and others that we love start needing more care than we know how to get them.

My mother moved into her first 55+ senior community when she was eighty-four. For ten years she lived an active, many might say enviable life. Unfortunately, year by year, month by month, day by day, her mind slowly deteriorated. She lived independently until she was ninety-four. It was a tumultuous ten years of good times/bad times, until her toxicity and descent into madness reached a point where she became both a risk to herself and to others.

Then one evening she accidentally put a (new) pan with rubber handles in the oven to broil some salmon (a favorite dish of hers) a few months after her 94th birthday. The rubber handles melted and the black smoke triggered her building's fire alarm. Her neighbors were fed up with her constant rants and tirades and crazy accusations and they complained to management enough for the 55+ community to use the accident as an excuse to evict her.

It was a little unfair because it was an accident that could have happened to anyone. But it wasn't entirely unwarranted. She was starting to become a hazard to herself and others and because she was so suspicious of everyone and so difficult to be around, no one was eager to be her friend, or be on a buddy system with her, to look after each other like many older residents living in the same building often do for each other.

Before I had to move her into her first professional, full-time senior facility, I was checking in on her just about every other day and talking with her on the phone often multiple times a day. Her well-being, specifically her mental well-being, had taken over my life. None of the mood stabilization drugs her doctors prescribed had worked. But with round the clock attendants and nurses that monitored her, did her cleaning, took care of her laundry, helped her get dressed, saw that she went down to eat breakfast, lunch and dinner with her neighbors, took her (new) pills and vitamins, and kept her distracted enough with group activities and outings, I felt confident my mother would be safe from herself and could maybe possibly be happy at least some of the time.

But that was another false hope.

In many ways, moving my mother into a fully assisted living facility was trading one set of problems for another.

I'll go into more about those challenges in the next chapter. The bottom line is that my stress did NOT go down. I thought it would go down. I expected it to go down. I told myself it would go down. But it didn't. The phone calls not only didn't abate, they increased. Because now they were coming from my mother AND the facility where she was living.

She was almost impossible to talk to or be around because in her deranged mind everyone, including me, was against her and constantly plotting to do her harm. But she still had her health. She was still dressing herself, eating three meals a day, didn't have any problems with incontinence and didn't need a walker to get where she was going. The stories about her life were starting to change though. The people and the places were getting mixed up and she wasn't catching it. The forgetfulness was just one more thing, in a seemingly never-ending heap of things, but at least she was safe and living in a nice place where there were multiple nurses 24/7.

The phone calls kept on coming though, and I didn't know what to do but answer them because when I didn't, the sense of dread about having to eventually call her back was in some ways worse than just getting it over with.

I didn't realize how much my mother's deteriorating condition had become my problem until I felt a shooting pain in my chest.

In late July 2018 I was at a lovely B&B in Flagstaff, Arizona on my way home from a business trip in beautiful and serene Sedona when my phone rang. My blood pressure had been spiking every time my phone rang for more than three years by then, but the sudden, sharp pain in my chest was a warning sign that even I couldn't deny. I was 215 pounds of raw nerve at that point, and in retrospect I should have known that a mini vacation to the Sonoran Desert was not going to cure me.

Fortunately that incident (more about it in the next chapter) turned out to be the wake-up call that I needed. I started dealing with my pent-up stress and seeking more help with my mother's constantly deteriorating condition. (More about how I did that in **Chapter 5 - How To Cope**)

Six months after that phone call, she was evicted again and I had to drop everything (again), this time to find a full-time memory care facility where she could live.

My mother turned 96 a few months after that. By that point her memory was failing rapidly and she was starting to have some mobility problems, although she refused to use a walker. The stories about her life she had told hundreds of times were all mashing together. Names and places and events were all mixed up and became interchangeable fragments. Her memories were like soup, indistinguishable from one another because they were so stirred together.

At that point she finally became the proverbial "sweet old lady" and she wasn't nearly as toxic as she had been before. I was glad I had lived to see her make that transition. It wasn't easy to watch though because she started losing the ability to speak, and then the once-graceful, beautiful dancer was confined to a wheelchair because she fell and broke her hip.

Fortunately, by then I was admitting to myself that the stress of dealing with my mother's condition had almost killed me and that for my own good, I needed to process and deal with everything that happened to her from then on with a certain amount of zen-inspired detachment.

After reading the rest of my book, I invite you to share the trials and tribulations, the wins and the successes, of your caregiving journey too. Visit my blog, **The Caregiving Project** (www.thecaregivingproject.com) to unburden, share, vent, ask questions, ask for advice, or find other caregiver related resources. I'm hoping that with the support of **Alzheimer's Nevada**, the **Lou Ruvo Center for Brain Research** and other regional and national organizations, The Caregiving Project will be able to co-create helpful podcasts with live call-ins and other features to build a community of support for caregivers no matter where they live.

CHAPTER 2

FIVE RULES FOR BEING AN EFFECTIVE CAREGIVER

Over the course of the fifteen years I watched my mother's descent into the murkier and murkier, deeper and deeper depths of dementia, and the past three when the classic symptoms of Alzheimer's came on strong and took over, I've discovered several hard truths of being a caregiver that I wish someone had shared with me back in the beginning when I first noticed my mother start to change into someone I no longer knew.

Some of those discoveries have been rather complex, such as those I discuss in **Chapter 3 - The Difference Between Dementia and Alzheimer's** and **Chapter 6 - Treatments and Medications.** Other discoveries, like what I discuss in: **Chapter 4 - What To Expect As A Caregiver, Chapter 5 - How To Cope With Being A Caregiver,** and **Chapter 7 - Making The Most of The Time That's Left** were more difficult.

But some of my discoveries, the basic, simplest ones, can be boiled down to what I call:

FIVE RULES
FOR BEING AN
EFFECTIVE CAREGIVER

These five easy-to-remember truths will prepare anyone who has to face the hard, cold realities of caring for someone afflicted with any sort of dementia. Whether it's Alzheimer's, Parkinson's, Vascular, or any other degenerative neurological disorder.

Although I discovered each one of these five rules the hard way — through my own personal experience — I know from talking with dozens of different doctors, nurses, activity directors, facility administrators, and hundreds of other sons, daughters, brothers, sisters, husbands, and wives, that they are wholly universal.

If you ever want to see a bunch of people nod their heads all at once, lay one of these five rules on a room full of people even remotely familiar with the challenges of dementia care, and I can almost guarantee they will all nod their heads in solemn, often silent, agreement.

Rather than try to rank them by order of importance though, I am going to present them in the order I realized them.

For me, the first one was the one that made me step back and look at my mother's decline from a broader perspective. But each has its own magnitude, relevance and importance at different stages of the caregiving journey, so which one resonates the most with you will probably depend upon where you are at in your caregiving journey.

RULE #1 -
No One Asks How YOU Are Doing

Your loved one is the one with the problem, right?

Yes. But your loved one's problem increasingly becomes your problem. Not just logistically, emotionally, or financially. But also in terms of your own health because of the incredible amount of usually buried stress that can build up.

Your loved one's problem can begin to affect your mental health, your spiritual health and ultimately, even your physical health.

This is the number one rule of caregiving I wish I could have known at the start of my caregiving journey. Or even in the middle of it—because it would have helped me better anticipate and deal with the stress I spent years suppressing.

When friends and extended family find out that you are caring for someone suffering from Alzheimer's, or any other form of disease really, they generally express their empathy by asking, "How's your mom?" or "How's your dad?" or more generally, "How are they doing?" every time they see you. There might be a platitude here and there along the lines of, "This must be so hard on you" but any focus on you the caregiver generally ends there.

As caregivers thrust into often very complex, very emotional, very stressful situations, we generally answer these questions by offering a knee-jerk, summarized account of the latest challenge, or the latest health emergency, or the latest manifestation of insanity exhibited by our loved one. We might even throw in a little humor to try to prove to them (and ourselves) that we're handling it okay.

Because our loved one is the patient, right?

It makes sense that they are the one under the microscope of analysis and problem management, right?

Well, yes and no.

Like our well-meaning friends and extended family, when WE typically forget to ask OURSELVES how we are doing, WE are ignoring a BIG part of our patient's fundamental care.

It's not our friends fault that they don't understand how stressful caregiving for a loved one can be.

It's not our family's fault either.

But it is our fault if we forget to check-in with ourselves along the way to make sure that WE are coping with the situation.

Studies have shown that over 60% of all caregivers develop a serious health condition of their own due to the psychological, emotional and physical stress of caring for a loved one.

Health professionals call it **Caregiver's Syndrome**, or sometimes, **Caregiver Stress**.

Symptoms in caregivers for loved ones with Alzheimer's or other dementia are typically exhaustion, resentment, anger or even sudden outbursts of rage. I'm embarrassed, but not too proud, to admit that I was so frustrated once after getting off the phone with my mother one time in 2013 that I threw a perfectly good, fully functioning cell phone against the wall in my office so hard it shattered into at least fifty pieces.

It felt great.

I regretted doing it almost instantly. But boy, did it feel great.

Another natural, but too often buried, emotion besides frustration that often causes Caregiver's Stress is soul-crushing guilt resulting from an inability to reverse or even just stabilize the effects of degenerative neurological diseases like dementia, Alzheimer's, Hodgkins, or others. The continuous struggle that comes with caring for a chronically ill patient, along with the tough medical decisions that have to be made and the financial challenges, causes stress to build up slowly, almost imperceptibly in caregivers, until it becomes ravenous and uncontrollable, eating us from the inside out.

I had all of those symptoms and more.

By the time I felt that shooting pain in my chest, I was having real trouble focusing on anything other than my mother's near-constant problems. I could barely work. I was drinking too much, watching too much TV, and generally desperate for just about any and all distractions. For a while, I took solace in civilization-building video games. They provided comfort because they proved beyond a doubt that I could make the right decisions to build, manage and maintain a thriving, healthy population in a world filled with a myriad of unpredictable threats and challenges. I was a level-10 player, which, subconsciously I think, proved to me that I knew what I was doing.

But whenever I would have a conversation with my mother it would often echo and reverberate in my head for hours, usually days, sometimes even weeks afterwards. I was constantly searching for the right explanation, the right line of reasoning that could help her escape from the deranged, haunted world of mixed up narratives, and anxiety fueled paranoia she was lost in. But I never could. No one could. But I kept trying—which kept adding to my stress that I kept on suppressing until I almost had a heart attack.

If WE don't make sure that we're getting all the help, advice, and shoulders to lean and cry on that WE NEED, it's not likely that anyone else will either. Because hey, we're not the patient, right?

But a caregiver must treat THEMSELVES like a patient too.

*Because a dead caregiver
is the worst caregiver of all.*

When I admitted to myself that my mother's ever-increasing decline was also affecting my health, I realized that was, in large part, because I had been so focused on making sure her world was as whole and complete as it could be. In doing that, in being there for her all the time, morning, noon and night, I lost sight of the fact that I needed to be making sure that MY WORLD was as whole and complete as it could be too.

And if it wasn't, that I needed help — or at the very least someone to talk to about it (see *Rule #5 - You Are Not Alone*).

But because no one else is likely to ask us how we are doing because we aren't the "real" patient, it becomes all the more important that we remember to check-in with ourselves and ask, "How am I doing?" and "What do I need to help me deal with this?"

I found that the best way to motivate myself to start taking better care of myself was to ask myself, "What would happen to my mother if I was no longer around to help her?"

RULE #2 -
They Forget, But You Don't

Apart from the logistical, medical and financial stresses that are often caused by the realities of different caregiving situations, patients with dementia also tend to make repeated, burning, extremely hurtful and mean accusations towards everyone around them.

These accusations are most often hurled at those who love them most and are trying to care for them.

In **Chapter 4 - What To Expect As A Caregiver** I am going to outline some of the incredibly hurtful, absolutely delusional things my mother said to me. But for now, I'm just going to say that the weeping sadness and dark pits of despair that caregivers are often forced to wade through with their loved one for hours and hours on end, day after day, week after week, and sometimes even year after year, often start to follow a pattern.

But just because these outbursts (might) become predictable, doesn't mean that they are any easier for the caregiver to deal with.

Because the person afflicted with dementia usually has the luxury of forgetting what they said immediately, or not long after, they said it.

This is especially true with Alzheimer's patients. (More about the practical distinction between dementia and Alzheimer's in the next chapter — it's very important and is something else that not enough people talk about!)

But as caregivers we DON'T have that same luxury of forgetting.

- Words and conversations can and will start to echo in a caregiver's head for hours or even days after they are spoken.

- I spent countless hours playing conversations with my mother over and over in my mind searching for a rational, or logical explanation, or the ever-elusive perfect counter-argument to alleviate her latest delusional outburst.

- We will drop everything and spend hours finding a solution for what seems to them like the most pressing problem on the planet, only to discover later they've completely forgotten about that particular problem and moved onto something even more dire. (Thus perpetuating the endless cycle of continuous woe and dread the dementia caregiver must contend with.)

The subtlety of this stressful pattern can and invariably almost always does take a very serious toll when, as a caregiver, we aren't aware of and don't <u>anticipate</u> or <u>prepare</u> for the emotional rollercoaster that is a caregiver's journey.

You are NOT going to be able to forget some of the mean, awful things your loved one with dementia is likely to say to you while they are in the depths of their disease.

Well-meaning friends and family will tell you that "you have to." You can try. But you will, I'm sorry to say, eventually fail.

You can try to bury it. But again, you will fail.

The echoes of those awful accusations will not only frustrate you, they will make you angry.

Eventually, after you've heard how horrible and diabolical and cruel you've been to them over and over and over again, they will even start to make you doubt yourself. Are you doing enough to help them? Probably. But it may not feel like they appreciate it one single bit.

Worse, they might even make you suspicious of the friends and family in your caregiving circle.

The only way I found that worked for me to get rid of this frustration and feelings of doubt was to confront them and process them.

Did I argue with my mother when she made her outlandish statements and accusations? Yes. Did it help? Not one single bit. Usually, it only perpetuated the argument.

For a while I tried ignoring them, or glossing over them. Out of desperation I tried laughing at them. But that proved to be the worst strategy of all because it just made her even more piss-mad.

Nothing worked. If I glossed over or ignored her outbursts, in her mind that just confirmed that what she had just accused me (or my wife, or her sister, or anyone else) of was true. If I addressed them and tried to convince her she actually had nothing to worry about, or that I would handle it so that she didn't have to, that caused her to spiral down to the bottom of some new, even worse despair.

My once amazing, awesome mother seemed to relish thinking up the meanest, cruelest thing she could accuse me of and then calling me either first thing in the morning, or at the most inconvenient time in the middle of my day, to try and devastate me with it.

Too often, it totally worked.

I can't even begin to count how many times she completely ruined my day with one of her cruel, toxic accusations. It took me a long time to take that power away from her. But finally I did. (I'll talk about how in **CHAPTER 5 - How To Cope With Being a Caregiver**)

They forget, but you don't may sound obvious and simplistic. But it's important to keep in mind when trying to understand the complex and emotional ways our relationships with our loved ones suffering from dementia will, inevitably, change.

RULE #3 -
Not Everyone Who Works In A Nursing Home Is A Saint

Far, <u>far</u> from it sometimes.

When I answered that phone call in Flagstaff that caused those shooting pains in my chest, I knew it was not my mother because I had assigned a specific ring to her number years earlier so that I could decide whether to take her call or not. I looked at my Caller ID and since it was from the facility where my mother was living at the time, I decided to take the call hoping it would be some good news from the doctor's visit I knew she had just had.

Surprise, surprise, it was not about her doctor's visit. It was one more countless last straw arriving right at the pinnacle of me and my wife feeling positive and optimistic about the future for the first time in years.

It was another nuisance paperwork request from a facility administrator who delighted in complicating other people's lives with her tiny, little shred of authority.

This woman was a real piece of work. She had repeatedly told me she had everything necessary to renew my mother's lease, but then she would call with "one more little thing." She knew my wife and I were leaving for a much-needed vacation. But in her petty little world it was the perfect opportunity to call me and demand that I bring a post-dated envelope that had come with one of my mother's financial statements, or she would begin eviction proceedings while my wife and I were out of the country.

This was a nice, relatively affordable, income-restricted facility here in Las Vegas that my mother had qualified to get into the year before and this woman herself told me the renewal was "just a formality" since absolutely nothing had changed with my mother's finances. In fact, my mother's meager retirement savings had gone down because the cost of her care had increased so much over the past year. She was actually MORE qualified to live there than she had been the year before because what little money my mother had wasn't even in the stock market. It was in low-yield, cash convertible municipal bonds to avoid risk, which meant that it hadn't appreciated at all.

My mother was well under the income threshold, but I was being made to jump through hoops simply because this woman got her jollies by making other people's lives miserable. I found out later I was not the only one she did this to and that she and the executive director of the facility, who walked around as if on rarefied air too, were the main reason there was such a high turnover rate with employees.

I felt crushed. Why was this woman doing this? Why was she making a difficult situation even worse? Why couldn't I have one week, hell, even just three days to myself without my mother going into some soul-crushing psychotic rage, or the facility where she was living making me jump thru crazy, unnecessary hoops just because they could?!!

It was then and there, staring at the serene, utterly peaceful view out the window from the second floor of the beautiful, historic Inn at 410 in downtown Flagstaff, Arizona that I realized this was the last straw ... almost ... for me.

Fortunately I had the presence of mind not to blow up. I tried to reason with her but it was useless. I knew right then and there I was the only one who had the power to make this straw the one that *didn't* break my back.

Instead, I made it the one that saved my life.

I agreed to her latest ridiculous demand. Then, I hung up the phone and finally admitted for the first time, out loud to myself, and to my wife who was sitting next to me with a worried look on her face, that I had a problem.

Aside from petty administrators who delight in making the residents, the primary caregivers of the residents, and even the other employees at a facility unnecessarily miserable, other things to watch out for in nursing homes or other eldercare facilities are:

- **THEFT** - my mother was robbed blind. Cash was stolen out of her purse, her clothes and directly out of her apartment. She didn't need any cash at the full-care facilities she was at but always felt safer with a little on her. The week I was forced to move her out of one facility into another, someone, and I have a pretty good idea who, stole her whole empty wallet out of sheer meanness. There wasn't a cent in it.

Not even in the tiny coin purse. But her driver's license was in it. Her Social Security and Medicare cards were in it. Her In Case of Emergency Card was in it.

- **THEFT** - jewelry. Every single one of my mother's 14kt, 18kt and 24kt gold necklaces was taken, not by other residents who conned her or tricked her out of them, but by specific nurses and attendants who checked in on her regularly and who she (and I and my wife) trusted. They stole ALL of her jewelry, even her emerald wedding ring, and left cheap costume jewelry in place of it so that on first glance, her bureau and dresser tops didn't look barren. Eventually though, even the costume jewelry was stolen.

- **THEFT** - clothes and even wigs! Right up until my mother was practically bedridden, she took great pride in how she looked. She dressed every single morning. For years on her own, and then with some assistance. She had nice things. Until she didn't. The nurses and facility administrators helped themselves to her dresses, leather jacket, and yes, even her wigs!

- **CAREGIVER PRO TIP #1** - whether your loved one is in a shared room or has their own private apartment at a facility, trust no one. They will smile in your face and deserve an Oscar for their selfless acts of compassion, but check the cart they wheel into your loved one's room. If it's got any drawers or compartments, or a heavy curtain around the legs, you should assume they have stuff hidden and tucked away on that cart that is not theirs. Bottom line, you cannot let your constantly confused or good-natured, absent-minded loved one have any nice things in an eldercare facility. If you do, check REGULARLY that they still have them. If you see anything missing report it immediately and then follow up on the report. But don't expect the missing items to suddenly be found. I reported things that went missing in my mother's apartment and when I followed up was told that I should have reported it. I did report it! Another thing to look out for is high staff turn over. Nurses, nurse practitioners, laundry, cleaning and food staff are notoriously underpaid at most care facilities. If you hear of anyone leaving, lock up your loved one's valuables and be sure you're the only one with the key or combination to the safe. If you hear of anyone who has recently left, do a thorough inventory, scream at the moon and re-read the first sentence of this Pro Tip.

- **FOOD** - If your loved one is on a special diet by doctors orders and that special diet is listed on your loved one's chart or in their file at a nursing home or eldercare facility, do NOT trust that the kitchen staff at the facility knows anything about it. My mother was supposed to be on a low-sodium diet. They swore to me she was on a low-sodium diet. Two weeks after I had to move her from one facility to the next, I noticed her ankles had swollen up into pillows and that her shoes weren't fitting anymore. I talked to the nurses. I talked to the doctor who checked on her once a week. They were all baffled. They blamed the new mood stabilizer prescription we were trying. Then one day my wife and I accidentally mis-timed our visit and arrived during lunchtime. So we sat with her while she ate. She felt bad we had come to take her to lunch (this was after the Alzheimer's had replaced most of the more toxic aspects of her personality) so she offered us bites of her food. Guess what? Super, SUPER salty!!! This may sound like isolated incompetence, or maybe even just laziness on the part of the staff where I happened to have my mother, but it's not. I've talked with dozens of other caregivers who have had the exact same experience with their loved ones at other facilities both here in Las Vegas and in many other cities too.

- **DRUGS** - I'm sure there are going to be some physicians and nurses, psychiatrists and other medical professionals who will read what I've written so far about my mother and her long struggle with psychosis and dementia and say that she should have been prescribed stronger antipsychotic and mood stabilizing drugs earlier. The fact is, my mother knew she had a problem early on and did seek out help in a bottle. First, to reduce her residual stress from living through the Northridge Earthquake and then during her recovery from her triple bypass. But nothing seemed to work. The drugs made her slightly less volatile and her mood swings less severe, but the side effects were long, morose bouts of depression. No "medicine" she could find in a bottle could replace a long walk along the beach, a laugh and a beer or two with friends and family, a rousing performance by the National Symphony Orchestra, or getting out onto a dancefloor.

- **CAREGIVER PRO TIP #2** - Beware of pill pushers. They are everywhere in the nursing home and eldercare landscape and they do NOT usually have your loved one's best interest at heart. Do your research. Watch out for side-effects. Each prescription has its own set and many doctors are happy to prescribe one drug to alleviate your loved one's depression or anxiety, and one or two others to try and control the side effects of the first one. All of these drugs wreak havoc on your loved one's thyroid and pituitary glands. (The pituitary gland controls the activity of most other hormone-secreting glands and for that reason is often called "the master gland.") I'll talk a little more about Treatments & Medications in **CHAPTER 6** but suffice it to say there are few, if any, magic answers in a bottle to depression, anxiety, Alzheimer's, or any other dementia that work better than a healthy, low-sodium, low-fat, balanced diet along with regular mental and physical stimulation.

No one is going to care for your loved one as much as you no matter how much you pay them. And it's a safe bet that many, if not most, of the staff at the nursing home or eldercare facility where your loved one is living are underpaid, so that unfortunate fact should be taken into consideration rather than ignored.

You have the choice of implicitly trusting everything they tell you.

Or, checking everything they tell you yourself and arriving at your own conclusions.

You need them to do their job because the stress and strain of providing full-time memory and physical care to someone, even if you think you have the time and space in your life to do so, cannot be overstated. It is a HUGE job and one that professionals, even semi-professional professionals, can do way better than you. But it is your job to help them do their job as well as possible, without becoming a victim in the process.

RULE #4 -
It's Going to Get Worse Before It Gets Better

I struggled long and hard with whether to include this rule or not. It was in my original draft that I wrote in the spring of 2019, but then I took it out that summer because I wanted the overall tone of this book to be supportive and positive.

I told myself I wanted this book to be more about the trials and tribulations that the caregiver of a dementia or Alzheimer's patient must face, rather than the ones their loved one must face.

But then my mother started falling.

The once-elegant ballroom dancer—who toured with Arthur Murray when she was in her 20s, and then returned to dancing later in life in her 60s and not only entered but won several competitions in the waltz and swing and the rumba (her favorite), and then moved west and fell in love with and won several competitions in country-western line dancing in her 70s, all the way up to when she was 80; this once-graceful person who walked up and down the first, second and third tiers of the Kennedy Center seating patrons several days a week well into her retirement—needed a walker just to get to the bathroom.

Witnessing that sad metamorphosis was just as difficult as the long, frustrating, stuck-in-the-bottom-of-a-well conversations I faced as a caregiver. The anger and stress of dealing with manipulative facility administrators, petty thieves, and incompetent, under- or over-paid pill pushers who care more about maximizing their revenue than addressing real issues of wellness sucks, too.

RULE #5 -
You Are Not Alone

There are A LOT of people in the United States, and the rest of the world, suffering from Alzheimer's and other forms of dementia. This means there are even more primary and secondary caregivers dealing with the challenges of the disease too. So the topic of aging and Alzheimer's is becoming more and more prevalent, both around our dinner tables and in our daily media barrage.

According to the Alzheimer's Association, there were 5.8 million people currently suffering from Alzheimer's in the United States in 2020. However, many in the health care industry feel that number is significantly understated because it does not include undiagnosed cases, nor does it include all forms of dementia. (*Alzheimer's is a type of dementia, but they are not the same—I will go into the differences between Alzheimer's and dementia in Chapter 3.*)

I both love and respect the work the **Alzheimer's Association** is doing. Their user-friendly website provides lots of valuable and surprising information. That said, based on the fact that my mother wasn't officially diagnosed with Alzheimer's until she was 95, I tend to agree that the estimate of just under six million people in the U.S. currently suffering from Alzheimer's is probably significantly understated, because the early manifestations of my mother's dementia emerged when she was 80. The disease posed significant problems for her, and me as her legal guardian and primary caregiver, long, long before she was officially diagnosed.

According to Pew Research, prior to the 2020 COVID-19 pandemic, there were just over 23 million people alive in the U.S. who were 75 or older (the so-called Silent Generation, plus the roughly 100,000 people left of those who were born before 1928—which Tom Brokaw aptly named the Greatest Generation, which was my mother's generation).

Add to the fact there are more than 72 million people in the United States between the ages of 56 and 74 (the Baby Boomers).

That's over 95 million people who are 56 or older! And that's just in the United States! There's a disconnect in the math for me when the Alzheimer's Association says that just under 6 million people have Alzheimer's in the U.S. right now, but that one in three seniors dies with Alzheimer's or some other form of dementia.

The bottom line is there are a lot of people with Alzheimer's or other forms of dementia. That number is expected to steadily grow in coming years, which means that every day there are more and more people forced into a caregiving role.

Globally, there are over 700 million people 65 or older!

So, caregivers have no reason to feel alone.

Caregivers do not have to put themselves under the tremendous pressure of solving all the problems and finding all the answers for their loved one's ever-deteriorating condition. Remembering that YOU ARE NOT ALONE makes you not only a better caregiver for your loved one but also a healthier caregiver for you and your immediate family too.

A lot of organizations, hospitals, and eldercare facilities are starting to focus more and more outreach and counseling programs on caregivers because they realize it makes their staff members' jobs so much easier to deal with a well-informed, less stressed-out caregiver or legal guardian.

I have been amazed at how much new information I see for caregivers, not only on the internet but also from organizations like the Alzheimer's Association. There is also much more community awareness and support coming from local 55+ and other senior-care facilities, libraries, and other organizations too.

*It's important for caregivers to talk
with and learn from each other.*

Even if your friends and family forget to ask how you're doing being the primary caregiver or legal guardian for someone suffering from Alzheimer's or other form of dementia, don't forget to ask yourself.

By being honest about what it is that we don't know and/or what we need help with, we can begin to reach out and find the support and the resources we need to overcome those challenges.

The good news is that support is out there! You just have to find what works for you.

A good place to start is the **Alzheimer's Association**, the **Dementia Society of America, AARP**, or **The Institute on Aging**. (*All their websites and many other resources are also listed in the Resource Section of my blog.*)

More and more information about aging and dementia is coming online and popping up in communities not just in the United States and Canada but also Europe and the rest of the world. So even though as a caregiver you might feel all alone, you absolutely are not!

CHAPTER 3

DEMENTIA OR ALZHEIMER'S?

Dementia is NOT a specific disease. But Alzheimer's is.

Within the medical profession, dementia is an umbrella term used to describe a category of different neurological disorders.

Different Types of Dementia

Presently, the Alzheimer's Association lists 11 different types of dementia.

1. Alzheimer's (the most common type of dementia) - forget-fulness & mood swings

2. Lewy Body Dementia (2nd most common) - hallucinations, severe depression

3. Vascular Dementia - hyper-anxiety, problems with judgement and reasoning

4. Frontotemporal Disorders - speech problems attributed to nerve loss in the brain

5. Parkinson's Disease - often associated with tremors and shaking

6. Huntington's Disease - a genetic disorder that causes uncontrolled movement

7. Normal Pressure Hydrocephalus - where the brain floods with fluid

8. Creutzfeldt-Jakob Disease - rare protein anomaly that progresses quickly

9. Posterior Cortical Atrophy - primarily causes vision problems

10. Korsakoff Syndrome - associated with prolonged misuse of alcohol

11. Mixed Dementia - which is a combination of two or more dementias

Other organizations, like the American Medical Association, the National Institute of Health, and even AARP have their own, evolving groupings and categorizations of dementia, but I've found that most of them are quite similar. This list from the Alzheimer's Association, and any list for that matter, is likely to grow in the future as researchers and scientists continue to study our brains, how they work, and especially how they don't work.

As I've already mentioned, I am not a doctor. So I am not going to attempt to make distinctions between each of these different types of dementia. However, based on my personal experience and the personal experiences many others have shared with me, I think it's safe to say my mother suffered from Mixed Dementia — specifically, a combination of Lewy Body Dementia, Vascular <u>and</u> Alzheimer's.

According to the National Institute on Aging, Mixed Dementia is becoming an increasingly common diagnosis that medical professionals in eldercare are using to describe patients because many symptoms overlap.

It makes sense. Not everyone who has dementia exhibits the same symptoms, in the same order, as everyone else. Sometimes delusional behaviour precedes forgetfulness. Sometimes forgetfulness precedes delusional behaviour. Sometimes dramatic mood swings, depression and/or hyper-anxiety comes after forgetfulness. Sometimes they manifest and exhibit prior to forgetfulness. Because I'm writing this book as a caregiver for someone who manifested a prolonged cognitive decline and a variety of different symptoms over many, many years, I want to be clear that:

Alzheimer's is a specific disease, dementia is not.

Although Alzheimer's and dementia are often used somewhat interchangeably, they are NOT the same thing. Not in terms of the patient's experience. And especially not in terms of the caregiver's experience.

As a caregiver, you will hear many medical and caregiving professionals, regardless of the specific type of dementia, refer to three basic stages of the disease. They are:

Early / Mild
Middle / Moderate
Late / Severe

This terminology is obviously rather generic and vague, but being familiar with it is useful when talking with others about your loved one's condition. They serve as jumping-off points for deeper discussions, planning, and caring on your particular journey as a caregiver.

A Deeper Look at Alzheimer's

Quick Facts

- Alzheimer's is the most common type of dementia currently being diagnosed. It is estimated to be the primary cause of somewhere between 60-80% of all dementia cases.

- Alzheimer's is a specific disease associated with how and where microscopic plaques and platelets accumulate in the brain.

- As of August 2020, it is estimated that approximately 6 million (6,000,000) people in the United States are currently suffering from Alzheimer's. Worldwide it is estimated to be over 50 million (50,000,000). And that's just Alzheimer's! Both of those numbers are somewhere between 20-40% higher when all forms of dementia are included!

- In the next 30 years, those numbers are projected to more than double.

- Roughly 80% of people suffering from Alzheimer's (according to current estimates) are over 75 years old. But that means a significant number, 20%, or one in five, are younger than 75. So just because your loved one isn't "old" yet, doesn't mean they might not be beginning to show signs of Alzheimer's or other form of dementia.

- Pre-Covid, the average life expectancy for both men and women in the United States was roughly 80 years old (it was less than 74 in 1980). That number might dip a little for a year or two, but once vaccines are widely distributed, it will likely continue to increase due to advances in medical technology and wellness.

- In the United States between 2000 and 2018, Alzheimer's as the primary cause of death for adults over 65 increased by almost 150%. (That means it doubled plus another 50%!)

- It is estimated that for every one Alzheimer's patient there are three (3) non-paid primary or secondary caregivers.

Alzheimer's is a word that at one point or another has been on the cover of just about every magazine I can think of. It's a recurring subject in news media not just in the United States, but also all around the world. Every country in the world is adjusting to their aging populations. Canada, Australia, England, France, Italy, Germany, Japan, China, Russia, and many other countries are pouring resources into how to manage and care for the explosive growth in their over-60 populations.

I always figured Alzheimer's was called Alzheimer's because of William von Wolfgang von Billy Joe Bob Alzheimer who researched brain stuff in aging adults 40,000 ga-zillion years ago at the University of Somewhere Far Away (UoSFA).

Turns out, I was close.

In 1901, a German psychiatrist named Alois Alzheimer identified the first case of what later became known as Alzheimer's disease in a fifty-year-old woman named Auguste Deter. He followed her case for five years until she died, and then by arrangement with the mental asylum where she had been living (yikes! right?) he was allowed to autopsy her brain with the help of several other surgeons. His autopsy revealed plaques and evidence of neurofibrillary tangles which still to this day are being studied and researched.

A colleague of his referred to his research as Alzheimer's Disease in 1910 and because the research was so groundbreaking and new, other studies about increasing forgetfulness, mood swings, depression and other behaviours associated with aging got lumped all together under the umbrella of his namesake research.

Thus, Alzheimer's was "discovered" — although, when the history of asylums and mental institutions is looked at, it's easy to argue the condition has been around for centuries. People dealt with all forms of cognitive and neurological disorders much less openly in the past. Even in my own lifetime, where I grew up on the East Coast, making a reference to a relative or someone that you knew who was "upstate" or "just back from upstate" was a not-so-subtle reference to a psychiatric ward. Over the years, it seems to have morphed in meaning to now mean time spent in a penitentiary. But even as recently as the 1970's and into the 1980's, the mental instability of relatives was rarely openly discussed.

Alzheimer's has become a general term not only for forgetfulness in older adults, but also for other mild to severe cognitive impairment. Many people use the term to describe mood swings, bouts of paranoia and depression, and other behaviour changes in their spouses, parents or other loved ones.

It's important to know that:

- Alzheimer's is NOT a normal process of aging

- since it is a progressive disease, it typically worsens over time

- unless another ailment outpaces it, it will, eventually, prove fatal

- life expectancy, depending on the person, can be anywhere from 3-20 years

The Different Stages of Alzheimer's

As I've already mentioned, the field of research and the terminology used to describe Alzheimer's and dementia is rapidly evolving. It is dynamically expanding in terms of diagnosis, treatment, and recommended care almost every single day. At the moment, many current professionals working with Alzheimer's patients reference NYU's Dr Barry Reisberg's framework for looking at the disease:

THE SEVEN STAGES OF ALZHEIMER'S

Stage One - Normal Outward Behaviour
(no visible signs)

Stage Two - Very Mild Changes
(lapses in remembering new things)

Stage Three - Mild Decline
(organization skills suffer, paranoia increases)

Stage Four - Moderate Decline
(financial management becomes a problem, old stories starts changing)

Stage Five - Moderately Severe Decline
(significant confusion and anxiety, lapses in personal care)

Stage Six - Severe Decline
(facial recognition declines, incontinence, high risk of falling)

Stage Seven - Very Severe Decline
(inability to communicate, eat, or swallow, death)

It's easy to fall down a rabbithole of information overload trying to diagnose where a loved one does or doesn't register on this scale. Doctors, nurses, pharmacists, other caregivers, care facility administrators, nurse practitioners and hospice workers are all eager to have that conversation though, and it's worth having no matter how painful it is to hear. It's important to have the right vocabulary to speak with them. But wrestling with the various and nuanced definitions of what is and isn't dementia, what is and isn't Alzheimer's, will only serve you, the primary caregiver and decision-maker, to a certain extent.

Practical Definitions of Alzheimer's and dementia

I do not disagree with the standard definitions of "dementia" and "Alzheimer's" generally used by those in the medical and eldercare fields.

However, I want to make a distinction between the two words because of how I experienced them in a practical sense, as a son trying to look after my mother in her later years.

Over the course of the 15-plus years I witnessed my mother's profound personality change and had to deal with her ever-worsening delusional outbursts, the chronic forgetfulness and decline most often associated with Alzheimer's didn't start to manifest until towards the end, about 3 years ago.

Which supports my feeling that she, like many other older people, was dealing not just with Alzheimer's, but with Mixed Dementia. Because the,

PRACTICAL DEFINITION of Alzheimer's is:
Someone you love is forgetful and it's becoming a problem for them.

and the,

PRACTICAL DEFINITION of dementia is:
Someone you love needs help but they are so toxic to be around it's becoming a problem for everyone, <u>including</u> you.

For over 10 years my mother was a walking, talking, fully functioning time bomb. She could turn combative towards anyone about any and everything at the drop of a hat. Such characteristics are more commonly associated with Lewy Body Dementia than Alzheimer's, but who really knows? Her delusional, venomous and completely random outbursts of rage and paranoia and despair slowly became the prevailing characteristics of her day-to-day personality, and that's all that really mattered.

To say those years were stressful on her is a huge understatement.

To say they were stressful on me is an even bigger one because during that entire time I thought that she was the one with the problem — not me! (See **Chapter 5 - How To Cope With Being A Caregiver** for more on this, because remember Rule #1 - Don't Overlook Your Own Health because a dead caregiver is the worst caregiver!)

When she started having trouble balancing her checkbook in 2014 I knew there was a problem because she had been a professional bookkeeper, controller and office manager for over 20 years. She not only had an accounting staff who reported to her, she worked on all the company's finance and tax issues with the outside accountants and auditors. She had balanced hundreds, if not thousands of accounts, for years and not only that, had taught many others how to do it too.

In the beginning she refused my help. Naturally she was proud and I respected that.

But when I found out she was calling her banks and blaming them for making mistakes on purpose (*because they hated her and didn't want her business anymore*), I finally insisted that she let me step in and take a look. By that time I already knew her ego was as fragile as an egg trying to perform a high wire act for some cruel, surreal circus, so I let her help me figure out how to make our case against the banks.

She resisted and shouted, arguing every step of the way while offering me a vast array of things to eat or that she could cook. Looking back, it was probably one of the more pleasant afternoons we spent together that year. Eventually I discovered that a balance hadn't been carried forward correctly in the prior year and once that error was fixed, I made sure that "together" we were able to account for every penny and balance to her current statement.

She was so relieved.

A huge burden had been lifted from her spirit. She was going to finally be able to get on with her life because she no longer needed to find a lawyer to sue them for "robbing" her.

Yaaaay!

Or so I thought. I went home with an inflated sense of calm and false hope that the dire, unrelenting phone calls were finally going to abate.

Two days later she found someone else to be absolutely furious and utterly depressed about. I think it was over a neighbor who was stealing her morning newspaper. I found out later it was a newspaper that had stopped coming because she hadn't renewed her subscription.

Of course, balancing the checkbook and renewing her newspaper subscription didn't matter in the least. Subconsciously, I probably knew that. Although I wasn't quite ready to admit it to myself yet at that point. As with other hurdles I had previously crossed with her, I remember feeling a great sense of relief and (temporary) satisfaction for solving a problem that had been causing her — and me because I had to hear about it over and over and over again — massive amounts of agitation for months.

I'm going to discuss more of these kinds of things in the next chapter, **What To Expect As A Caregiver**, but I'm mentioning them here because it exemplifies the difference between dementia and Alzheimer's that I want to make.

Not only was my mother unable to express any gratitude for solving her problem, she STILL blamed the bank on some level for causing the out-of-balance situation even after I gently showed her how transposing two numbers on a check she had written months earlier had been the cause.

Despite being presented with the facts AND having her problem solved, her delusion that the bank had "wronged" her still persisted in her mind. There was nothing I could do other than stop trying to convince her otherwise.

The difference between being forgetful and being delusional is huge.

As I learned the hard way, making that distinction informs the best treatment options for going forward. It's easy to see that now. But when I was in the thick of it, when the endless, agonizing, despair-filled phone calls were raining down on me practically every single day, the coping mechanism I used was to solve each problem for her one by one as they arose.

Of course, no matter how much I did or how hard I tried, I was never solving the real problem. Never for very long at least.

From 2014 on, at age 91, my mother began exhibiting more and more of the generally acknowledged signs of Stage 3 Alzheimer's. Although she became even more delusional over the course of the next three years, she was able to live independently, pay her bills on time, cook, clean her apartment, shower, dress herself and go on outings with the active, 55+ senior community where she was living up until she was 94 years old.

Ninety-four years old!!

She ran, okay walked, circles around people ten, even fifteen years younger than her up until that point.

But, despite her physical health, her short-term memory was rapidly beginning to fail and she was becoming a danger to herself and others. Diagnostically she was probably moving from Stage 4 of the disease to Stage 5, so I moved her into a fully assisted living facility in 2017 where daily activities, bi-weekly shopping, sightseeing excursions, meals, maid and laundry service and other services were available. It helped. But it didn't help as much as I had hoped it would.

No matter what I, they, or anyone else did, no matter how often I called or went to see her, no matter how many times my wife and I took her to lunch, or dinner, or picnics with our dog that she dearly (most of the time) loved, my mother continued to be combative and argumentative and generally difficult for any and everyone to be around.

The person who had always made friends easily most of her life was not making friends anywhere anymore. Instead of decreasing, the dire, daily phone calls from the bottom of whatever new deep, dark well she had crawled into in her mind actually increased because now they were causing the nurses and facility administrators to call me multiple times per week, sometimes even multiple times per day, too.

That was the dementia.

She started repeating herself in the same conversation that year. That, to me, in my practical experience anyways, was the real start of her Alzheimer's. That's when her memory began to fall off the proverbial cliff. Within a year, she was in Stage 5 and the stories, names and places of her youth and younger days were all jumbled together.

Fortunately, as her memory faded her mean-spirited rage at everyone and everything around her began to fade too. The bursts of rage lessened to the point where the stereotypical, sweet, forgetful old lady started to become the prevailing characteristic of her day-to-day personality.

This change in her personality made her easier to deal with in one respect. By the time she was 95, she began to have more serious mobility issues. One of the recognized symptoms of Alzheimer's is when the motor coordination centers of the brain begin to be affected. However, one of the side effects of Lexipro (and other marginally effective mood stabilizing drugs) causes balance issues too. In less than 6 months, she went from needing a cane to walk to the dining area in the facility to needing a walker to stand up.

Her overall health and mobility and speech took a dramatic nosedive over the course of the next year. In 2019, three months before my mother turned 96, she needed to be moved into a secure, full-time memory care facility. The incontinence started (a common Stage 6 symptom) and that summer, the elegant, award winning dancer who was my mom started falling.

Was it because of the Alzheimer's?

Was it because of the drugs?

Was it a combination of both?

The next question a caregiver, or even just someone who cares, needs to ask themselves is: **Does it really matter?**

For me, at that point it was a name-the-poison situation. The fact that my mother was falling became more important than the reason she was falling.

I had no control over her disease and I was between a rock and a hard place with her meds. I believe her doctors were as honest with me as they could be.

But doctors do not fully understand dementia and many of them don't even agree with each other.

So, where does that leave you the caregiver?

The answer is, on your own to decide.

Because not only does Alzheimer's and other types of dementia affect different people differently, different drugs affect different people differently too. The only thing researchers know for sure is that the plaques and platelets that build up in the neural pathways of the brain because of Alzheimer's, and the excess proteins associated with Lewy Body Dementia, all affect and compromise each and every brain differently.

One of the things that makes degenerative neurological diseases like Alzheimer's, Parkinson's and others so challenging is that many medical professionals prefer to talk about the causes of the disease while caregivers are forced to deal with the symptoms of the disease, not the causes.

Cures for all forms of dementia, including Alzheimer's, are yet to be discovered. But, there is some promising research being done. Some studies have even shown that some activities and diets can delay the onset of many dementia symptoms.

But time will and does catch up with all of us eventually. After breaking her hip falling out of bed over Thanksgiving weekend in 2019, and after battling the manifestations of her neurological decay for over 15 long years, two month's shy of her 97th birthday my mother started having trouble swallowing and stopped eating. One month later, as Covid exploded around the world, she finally got better and transitioned to a higher place.

Alzheimer's, respiratory failure and heart disease were all listed on her death certificate. Which one actually killed her doesn't matter to her and it doesn't matter to me either.

Telling the Two Apart

Alzheimer's Disease is a form of dementia.

So why two different words? Are they different, or not?

No.

And, yes.

Although many in the medical field refer to the symptoms of Alzheimer's and dementia together, by their own definitions the symptom sets vary and they can exhibit multiple different ways in real life.

Maybe medically they are similar because based on current research they both involve clogging of the neural pathways of the brain in one way or another by the amyloid plaques and peptides that Alois Alzheimer Frederich Lewy identified back in 1906.

But outside the umbrella definitions used by medical professionals, the media and sometimes even our family or friends, as a caregiver I've observed significant differences between the characteristics of the two diseases.

Again, that might partly be explained by a more accurate diagnosis of Mixed Dementia for my mother than the simple Alzheimer's one that was eventually put on top of all her charts and medical records. But the fact of the matter is, that is what happened and so for the sake of brevity, I'm pointing it out simply because it's likely to happen for other patients and caregivers in the future.

As I have done already (and will continue to do throughout the rest of this book) I am going to make distinctions between the forgetfulness associated with Alzheimer's and use dementia to refer to other symptoms and behaviours associated with growing older, because as a loving caring adult child trying to do what's best for an aging parent, dealing with issues of memory loss was very different than dealing with open hostility and the many, very separate issues that came with it.

I'm not making these distinctions to challenge the medical establishment or advocate that they change their terminology or definitions. I actually think that as a whole, the medical community is doing an excellent job of embracing and trying to learn from, rather than ignore, health issues related to the longer life spans of our species.

Yes, there are similarities:

- Both can begin to manifest after traumatic catalyst events.

- Both can become increasingly debilitating over time.

- Both require more and more diligence and attention in terms of caregiving.

I'm making these distinctions because, like I said:

- Dealing with forgetfulness is one thing.

- Dealing with hissing mad at everyone and everything all the time is something else entirely.

In discussing, and more importantly NOT discussing (in the beginning), my experiences with others dealing with aging parents, I learned about the more subtle, but no less profound differences between what's commonly referred to as Alzheimer's and what's much less commonly (but very accurately) called dementia.

For better or worse, our media has embraced and our society has accepted the term "Alzheimer's" as both the clinical diagnosis and generic reference for many behaviors associated with growing older.

The generic term has helped increase overall awareness of the disease (some argue national epidemic) but:

there are other symptoms besides forgetfulness so it is not an entirely accurate label.

So again, I'm writing this book from the perspective of a loving caregiver rather than a medical one. As I already have done, I will continue to make distinctions between Alzheimer's and dementia because dealing with issues of memory loss is different than dealing with hostility.

Very separate issues are involved. Especially for the caregiver.

However, rather than try to invent a new way to label or re-define Alzheimer's, I'm going to perpetuate the association of Alzheimer's with forgetfulness in order to use the term "dementia" to refer to the more hostile and toxic characteristics that can manifest in the people we love.

Many of the distinctions between forgetfulness and what could be called behavioral dementia became apparent to me, in part, because I watched my mother's increased hostility coincide with her younger sister's increased forgetfulness. Her sister never became as mean-spirited and toxic to be around as my mother did. But ironically, my mother didn't begin to exhibit forgetfulness until ten years AFTER her younger sister did.

My mother was in her early 80's. Her sister was in her early to mid 70's.

In some respects their paths were similar. But in many others their journeys were quite different because my mother pushed everyone away from her and her sister did not.

CHAPTER 4

WHAT TO EXPECT AS A CAREGIVER

Alzheimer's is the most common form of dementia and therefore there is more known about it than the others, except maybe for Parkinson's and Hodgkins which are statistically very rare. Although I would be hesitant to equate the defined stages of Alzheimer's with the stages patients with one or more of the other types of dementia experience, in my mother's case, there were some similarities in terms of the increasing severity of her symptoms. (As previously noted though, in my mother's case, her breaks from reality, paranoia, rage, and depression preceded the onset of her forgetfulness by at least ten years.)

What's Going To Happen

I listed the generally agreed upon Stages of Alzheimer's in the previous chapter, rather than here, because how a caregiver experiences their loved one progressing through those stages is not identical to their patient.

The first two stages, typically referred to as Normal Outward Behavior and Very Mild Changes, are hardly noticeable to the person with the early onset of the disease, or those around them. They are useful in that they can be detected on a PET scan though, and for that reason alone I am mentioning them because it is possible that early detection could prove to be important to slowing, or perhaps even neutralizing the build-up of those nasty, sticky proteins and platelets in the future.

Stage 3 is often when symptoms of the "Mild Decline" associated with Alzheimer's become noticeable though. Generally the ability to form new, short-term memories is the first warning sign that a loved may be experiencing the onset of Alzheimer's. Trouble parking their car is another typical warning sign. Again, for me it was my mother's dramatic break from reality over Christmas in 2004 when she got it stuck in her head that everyone hated her and was laughing at her and was embarrassed by her and blah, blah, blah. Her memory was fine. But her grip on reality was beginning to slip. She also started using the f-word for the first time ever in her life.

Stage 4 is when symptoms of "Moderate Decline" become evident. For the Alzheimer's patient this can be frequently forgetting what day or month or even year it is, forgetting to pay their bills on time, or ordering from a menu (i.e., looking for the cheeseburgers on a menu for a Chinese restaurant) and having difficulty driving. For someone with Mixed Dementia who might not be forgetting anything yet, it can be more frequent bouts of hyper-anxiety, paranoia, blame and hurtful accusations.

Stage 5 is what is called "Moderately Severe Decline" and this is typically when things begin seriously affecting your loved one's life and your own. For the Alzheimer's patient, this can involve the beginning of mobility issues, getting lost in their own neighborhood, remembering what floor they live on if they live in an apartment building or eldercare facility, being able to dress or feed themselves properly and incontinence problems. For the mixed dementia patient, it can mean the sudden onset of all the Stage 4 and Stage 5 Alzheimer's symptoms, along with near constant paranoia, distrust of everyone around them, and physically lashing out at others.

The fact that Stage 6 is what is called "Severe Decline" probably comes as no surprise to anyone. For the Alzheimer's patient this typically includes chronic mobility issues including falling, near loss of memory, recognizing faces but forgetting names of loved ones, mistaking one person for another, and getting ready to go to a job they retired from many years ago. In my mother's case, as with most Mixed Dementia cases I've spoken with others about, this stage brought a welcomed lessening of her toxic rage and constant paranoia and hyper-anxiety, but the dramatic onset of the symptoms of Stage 6 Alzheimer's.

The last stage, Stage 7, "Very Severe Decline" usually includes, for both the Alzheimer's patient and those patients challenged with Mixed Dementia, the fading of the ability to walk, eat, and sit up on their own, along with trouble breathing and swallowing even liquids. This is the stage where doctors begin recommending feeding tubes, ventilators and other invasive medical procedures to keep the body alive because the brain has basically been so completely clogged with those sticky plaques and platelets that it has become unable to function.

Definitely make sure that you have said your good-byes before Stage 7 because your loved one will not be able to hear you or recognize you or speak to you by then.

What'll You'll Hear

As I discussed in the previous chapter, there is a huge difference between dealing with someone who is forgetful and someone who is delusional.

The delusional patient is likely to say the most hurtful and mean things that they can think to say to their caregivers. Especially those who love them the most.

My mother's delusions prompted accusations of:

- Being embarrassed by her

- Laughing at her behind her back

- Talking about her behind her back

- Conspiring with others to make her feel bad

- Wishing her harm

- Plotting to do her harm

- Hiring a hitman to kill her

- Wanting to pick her up to take her to lunch so that I could run her over with my car and make it look like an accident

- Training my golden retriever to attack her

- Stealing her money

- Working with her financial advisor of 30 years to forge fake account statements and sending them to her in the mail to make her think I wasn't

- Conspiring with my (long dead) father to come "get her" some night

- Hating her

- Wishing she was dead

- Hoping she would die

- Telling the doctors that performed her triple bypass in 1995 to let her die

- Being mad at them for not letting her die

- Lying to her (about any and everything)

- Plotting with her sister against her

And a whole host of other horrible, awful things, not one of which was true.

She would repeat them and change them up and intermingle them and lay them on me at 2 o'clock in the afternoon when I was at work, or 8 o'clock in the morning when I was having breakfast, or 6 o'clock in the morning when I was on vacation.

On top of all these venom fueled accusations that she would periodically start hurling at me for no reason, there were countless other calls where she would beg me to hire a hitman to kill her, "do her a favor" and blow her brains out, give her a gun so that she could end it all, put a pillow over her face "and end it," push her in front of a bus, and countless other morbid requests that I've pushed from my brain.

There was a period of time, I would say about five years before the Alzheimer's started really kicking in and shutting down her brain and her body just after she turned 95, that I was very concerned that she was borderline suicidal. I blame the "mood stabilizers" and anti-psychotic meds she was on as much as I do her dementia, but fortunately, her lingering Lutheran faith and me reminding her that suicide was a mortal sin, prevented her from doing anything to seriously harm herself.

I told her people who kill themselves come back in their next life with extra burdens to bear and that stuck with her for a long time. It actually usually cheered her up because she'd laugh and say something along the lines of "Well I sure don't want more burdens the next time around than I did this time" or something like that. The idea never prompted her to fall down a well of despair and recount some hard story from her past either.

Maybe in some strange way, it reminded her deep down what an amazing life she had had.

There is no rational argument you can use to calm a seriously delusional person. There is nothing you can say. Or promise. Or even do to demonstrate that you are there to help them and support them and see that they are comfortable and safe and happy.

Nothing.

Forget it.

Go ahead and try.

Then come back to this section and read it again.

The only defense a caregiver for a toxic dementia patient has for the mean, hurtful, completely baseless and outrageous accusations that will be hurled at them is:

1. take it

2. argue with it

3. or, process it

I'll talk about the best option of those three in the next chapter **How To Cope With Being A Caregiver.**

The Stages of Being A Caregiver

I believe that understanding the Seven Stages of Alzheimer's as currently defined and generally agreed upon can help guide in planning for the care of a parent, relative or dear friend suffering from the disease.

Looking at the stages of the dementia and the escalating demands from a caregiving perspective is more important than understanding what your loved one will potentially experience.

That's one of the main things I wish someone had told me when I first started on my caregiving journey. It would have alleviated so much stress and frustration and feelings of hopelessness.

Fortunately I did discover them about midway into my journey. They were helpful, although they were just words on a page until I experienced them. "Likely to experience repeated bouts of depression or extreme paranoia" didn't sound like my steady, rational, always able to laugh at her own mistakes mother.

It wasn't her.

But it did become her.

So although my mother did step through all seven stages of Alzheimer's, it's important to distinguish that:

the stages the dementia patient will go through are <u>not</u> the same benchmarks the caregiver will experience on their journey.

For someone caring for an Alzheimer's or dementia patient, whether it's on a full-time basis or a part-time basis, I believe they experience only three stages.

THE THREE STAGES OF BEING A CAREGIVER

Stage One - Denial
(distinguished by increasing amounts of buried stress)

Stage Two - Forgiveness
(distinguished by frustration and a sense of urgency)

Stage Three - Release
(distinguished by making a plan and surrendering to the path it takes)

Denial

Like the old saying goes, "Denial ain't just a river in Egypt."

Not surprisingly, it (denial) starts in the beginning. It lasts as long as the caregiver is willing to float along on its gentle, blissful current. The hope that happier times aren't in the rearview mirror flows from day to month to year.

It usually is traumatic for everyone involved when the power dynamics of the parent-child relationship begin to flip over to the child.

When a child becomes the primary advisor, protector and sometimes even provider for one or both of their parents, or any other loved one, the dynamics and patterns of previous communication methodologies change. The roles of provider, advisor, and coach flip.

But often not without acrimony and despair and heartfelt helplessness.

Just as our communication evolved from parent-child to parent-teen to parent-young adult to parent-mature adult, when our parents begin experiencing the ravages of old age, our communication evolves one more time as the power dynamic shifts from the parent to the child. It can be a very challenging process though.

- The bottom of the older person's self-esteem falls out

- Their sense of self-worth and their confidence in their own self-reliance crash

- They may not be aware that they resent any or all forms of help, yet they do

- The shift in the power dynamic can aggravate existing challenges that the caregiver is already dealing with

- The added responsibility of caring for an aging parent can put stress on the caregivers' marriages

- Old jealousies and competitiveness with other siblings can get stirred up

As communication breaks down, as more and more get-togethers and conversations end in an argument rather than resolution, stress increases on all sides.

Like a covered pot of water on a flame, stress eventually boils over.

And, often, it becomes just too much to think about at the moment so a let's-deal-with-one-problem-at-a-time approach becomes the default coping mechanism.

That was pretty much the route I took. I solved one problem at time for her for almost fifteen years until that strategy almost killed me.

The first year my mother started exhibiting signs of her dementia I knew her personality was changing but didn't know how to deal with it except by trying to maximize the good times and taking other things as they came. For an eighty year old she was doing great. Living on her own, shopping, cooking and cleaning for herself, while maintaining an active social life. She went to museums, she flew back and forth across the country by herself to visit relatives, she even packed up and moved across the country back to D.C. on her own with zero help from me. Then she packed everything up all by herself again a year later and moved to Las Vegas after visiting my wife and I after we moved there from southern California.

Over the course of the next ten years, the long, lamenting, pits of despair phone calls increased in frequency from every other month or so to pretty much several times a week. But she was still living on her own, going everywhere and anywhere she wanted on various senior transport options and even flying back and forth across the country by herself once or twice a year to visit her sister in either New York or Florida.

She hated doctors in her later years and pretty much refused to go see any until she got a viral infection and had to be hospitalized for a week. Many of the doctors at St. Rose fawned over her and marvelled at how well she was doing for a woman close to ninety. I got a few of the ones she seemed to like to talk with us about mood stabilizing options to address her increasingly frequent bouts of severe depression. But after politely listening to them and agreeing to let them write her a prescription, she turned on them with the venom of a rattlesnake the moment they were out of the room, labeling them all "pill pushers" and me a "terrible, rotten son" for even suggesting she ever struggled from radical mood swings or depression.

Unfortunately, I made the mistake of not pressing the issue. I got the prescription filled but she refused to ever take any of the pills.

The next three years after that were pure hell. Especially for me. Because it was around that time that she started having the luxury of forgetting whatever mean, awful, purposely hurtful thing she had said the last time we spoke. Our conversations echoed around in my brain for days, sometimes weeks at a time. Every time the phone rang, I dreaded that it might be her.

By that time I was no longer in denial that my mother had a problem. I was however still in denial that her problem was causing me health problems.

Finally, a full thirteen years after she first started exhibiting signs of delusional paranoia and thinking up the meanest possible thing she could think to say to me or anyone else around her, she got evicted from the 55+ community where she was living. The fire she accidentally started in her kitchen by putting a fish grill with rubberized handles into the oven was an honest, easy mistake just about anyone could have made. But our relationship had deteriorated to the point where I could barely talk to her anymore so I knew how difficult it had to be for the activity director and other administrators at the facility where she was living. The fact they considered her a threat to herself and the other tenants was not anything I even tried to argue with because I knew it was true.

They helped me get my mother into an affordable sister property in North Las Vegas that was a fully assisted-living facility with 24/7 on-call nurses, three meals a day, cleaning and laundry services, an active community events calendar, and even a nice view out her own private apartment.

Great! Finally! Problem solved I thought.

But no. The lamenting, pit of despair phone calls got worse and even more frequent. Sometimes eight, ten times a day starting as early as 5:30 in the morning. Fortunately, I finally had the luxury of knowing that she was safe and that other people were taking care of her. I didn't always have to take her calls anymore out of fear she had fallen or was hurt, but she was increasingly impossible to engage on anything other than a super toxic, venom-filled level about delusional convictions that if I didn't agree with I was automatically in on, and deserved any and all forms of verbal abuse she could think up to heap onto me. I went from trying to talk with her every day, to two or three times a week, to once a week, to once every other week. At first, either I, or my wife and I together, tried to visit her and take her out somewhere nice every other week. But nothing we did helped. She was constantly furious at everyone all the time. She seemed to save most of her wrath for me, which I joked was actually good because it meant she wouldn't antagonize and alienate the people being paid to take care of her. Ultimately this was just more of what I call my denial phase because although I clearly knew she had a problem, I still wasn't admitting to myself that I had a problem, too.

I thought I was coping by blocking her number when the phone calls got to be too many. I blocked her number for days, sometimes a week at a time. Once I forgot I had blocked it and had two whole weeks of not hearing the distinctive ringtone I had assigned her. I'm embarrassed but not too proud to admit that it was pure bliss — even though it was accompanied by an undeniable (stressful!) sense of dread about the mental holiday from her being too good to last.

Unfortunately, one of the administrators at the new place, I've mentioned her before already, was someone who was drunk with the little bit of power she had to complicate people's lives. Just as I was reducing the amount of time I was spending on the phone in pointless, hyper-toxic arguments with my mother about ridiculous delusional assumptions and accusations, nuisance paperwork requests started coming in on top of bi-weekly medical consults and incident reports from the activity directors.

I finally couldn't deny that my mother's problem was my problem any longer.

Forgiveness

It was actually really easy to forgive my mother. Intellectually I knew it was the disease, not her, making her say and do the things she was saying and doing. Applying that knowledge to what I knew emotionally in my heart, that I still loved my mother and cared for her and had been doing everything I could for her, made forgiving her for the things she had said and the demands she had put on me over the years quick and easy and painless.

It took a little longer to forgive myself for needing to take the time to back away and heal so that I could be there for her in the future (when, as it turned out, she <u>really</u> needed me to be healthy, present and clear-headed).

The effects of realizing that I was angry and frustrated and feeling hopeless about her deteriorating condition were almost instantaneously positive though. Like drinking a tall glass of cool water after hiking outside in the desert where I lived. Practicing a little scream therapy underwater in my friends' pools and out in the wild expanses of Death Valley and other parts of the Mojave Desert really helped too.

For me, expressing and letting out my frustration gave me the bandwidth to better assess the overall situation, both my mother's and mine.

I knew that things were likely to keep on deteriorating for her and that eventually she would probably need more care. I remembered myself as a young boy visiting my grandmother when she was in her nursing home and hoped that would never become my mother's fate, but began to accept the possibility. It's a good thing I did too, because it happened sooner than I expected. Less than six months after getting that call in Flagstaff that almost sent me over to the other side, my mother was deemed too unstable to stay where she was and I had to move her into a full-on, locked down, memory care facility.

Fortunately it was about half the distance from our home as her old place so I was happy for the little things. The new place had its own set of struggles (more about that in **CHAPTER 6 - Care Facilities and Treatment Options**) but my mother's toxic outbursts and paranoia had all but disappeared and now it was her physical health that was becoming the predominant thing she needed looked after.

I forgave the old place for robbing her blind. I forgave the administrator and her boss for being such petty human beings. I forgave myself for not having the presence of mind to put my mother's valuables, especially her beautiful emerald wedding ring, in a safe.

I knew I needed to be ready for the next thing, whatever it was going to be, and so I finally started preparing myself for it, instead of dreading it.

Release

Fortunately, I had developed a pretty good spiritual practice by that point and I started applying many of the New Thought principles my wife and I were exploring into my daily life. For me, meditating every morning helped heal my old wounds and lower my blood pressure. Michael Beckwith's book "Life Visioning" and May McCarthy's book "The Gratitude Formula" basically changed my life.

For the first time in years I actually had faith the future was going to be brighter. That good things were on the horizon. Not just in some vague future, but next month, next week, tomorrow, later today.

I started believing that the next time the phone rang it was going to be good news. That it wasn't going to be the facility where my mother was living. She lost the ability to use her cell phone, so the woe-filled calls from the bottom of the well stopped. When I picked up the phone it started being friends from college, or my friends in our wine club.

I started believing things not only were going to get better but that they already were better and guess what? It turned out they were!

It's not that there weren't any dark days during this period. There most certainly were. The first time my mother fell she bruised her face and gashed her head against a piece of furniture. Due to a mix up at the facility where she was living, I didn't even know about it until I got a call from the hospital five days afterwards asking when I was going to come pick her up.

The fourth time she fell she broke her hip and had emergency hip surgery the day before I was having a tricky patch of melanoma removed from under my eye. We both spent December 2019 recovering. I could have looked at it as huge hurdle and bad timing. But actually, in an odd way it was one of the last things we got to do together. I was whacked out on pain meds so it wasn't much of a challenge to sit with her in her dark room while she was whacked out on hers. (My wife Laura was the true saint in that situation because she had to drive me there and back and try to make sense of both my ramblings and my mother's!)

I did have, fortunately, the good sense to thank my wife and tell her how much I appreciated what she was doing for me. The whole experience, instead of being a terrible challenge, actually brought us even closer together because I wasn't resisting anything anymore. My mother pointed at the ghosts of my grandfather and grandmother and many of my favorite aunts and uncles in her recovery room. My mother was where she wanted to be and so was I.

For my mother there was a slow burn with her dementia. It came on slowly and lasted many, many years … like a piece of lost stardust descending into the horizon searching for a place to land. Slowly she disappeared until she was gone and all that was left was my memory, not hers.

I surrendered to that inevitable fate, but I'm glad I did manage to experience the forgiveness stage with her, and especially the very therapeutic release stage because it gave me closure. Closure that I wouldn't have had if I had kept on denying that she wasn't going to get better. Closure that I wouldn't have had if I didn't make the effort while she was still alive to forgive her, forgive the disease and forgive those who took advantage, or tried to take advantage of her situation. Getting to that stage of knowing that it was all going to be okay, without knowing how, made my journey as a caregiver easier when it finally came to an end.

CHAPTER 5

HOW TO COPE WITH BEING A CAREGIVER

The best way I found to cope with the stress of being a caregiver for a loved one suffering from dementia was to first admit that I was a caregiver and secondly to admit to myself that it is incredibly challenging.

One day I was describing how my mother had torpedoed my day by some crazy thing that she had said to me and a sympathetic friend who was in a similar situation said to me, "She isn't your mother anymore." Those five simple words instantly allowed me to give myself permission to start building a protective, emotional wall between me and the person I loved but didn't know anymore.

I had by that time already started attending a few caregiver's support groups at senior centers here in Las Vegas. I knew that my frustration with my mother for saying the things she said to me was the same frustration others in my situation felt towards their loved ones, too. It was good to know that I wasn't alone in what I was feeling. But I didn't need grief counseling. The phone calls were still a constant part of my life. The mood stabilizing medicine my mother was (supposedly) taking wasn't working. I needed a strategy for processing a problem that didn't seem to be getting any better or showing any signs of going away.

Although those support groups generally advocated taking a forgiveness approach to dealing with that frustration, I found that what worked far better for me was admitting and expressing my feelings out loud and, at first, pretty much to anyone who would listen.

As I hope that I've already made clear, I loved my mother very, very much. I respected her for all that she had accomplished in her life and I valued how much she encouraged me to follow my dreams and lead a positive, confident life. But she was not the same person I had loved and admired and respected my whole life anymore. The accumulation of sticky platelets in her brain had caused her to morph into someone else entirely different.

She was still my mother. But at the same time, she was so NOT my mother too.

I'm sure this will no doubt offend and shock some people, but I wasn't able to process the anger, and confusion and helplessness I was burying about my mother's ever-increasing toxicity until I started calling my mother a bitch. Not directly to her face, but in reference to her. As in, "my mother's a bitch" or more specifically, "my mother's a f-ing bitch." It helped immensely. Saying those words was so much more cathartic than throwing my cell phone against a wall and smashing it, or spending hours playing video games or Sudoku, or at the sportsbook to take my mind off my mother's latest, or pending, meltdown.

Ironically, once I started openly expressing my feelings this way to process them I found that I was not alone. Not at all. Although other sons and daughters didn't express their frustrations with their loved one's Alzheimer's or dementia in the exact same words all the time (many did though), my raw frustration provided them with an opportunity to express their pent-up, pushed down, buried feelings too.

By setting the bar so low, I noticed that I started providing others with a starting point to process their feelings. Friends and acquaintances started telling me that I needed to write a book. Other caregivers started coming to me for advice or just to talk. I joked about starting a workshop or seminar for caregivers here in Las Vegas and had numerous people ask me where they could sign up for it.

I told a psychologist friend of mine that I was considering creating a seminar and having a section in it where I tweak Arthur Janov's Primal Scream Therapy from the 1970's to use as a tool to vent frustrations for caregivers. She told me that the previously marginalized therapy (John Lennon and Yoko Ono were big fans of it when it first came out so it got laughed at by journalists at the time) is actually making a bit of a comeback these days.

It turns out that recent studies of the brain have shown that expressing frustration by screaming something about it stimulates a chemical reaction that creates a dopamine and endorphin hit that is similar to the one we get when we exercise.

When I (finally) took my friend Stephen Murray's advice in February 2019 to write a book about my experience as a caregiver for a loved one suffering from Alzheimer's and I mentioned it in casual conversation to other friends, over half a dozen speaking engagements presented themselves me in the first month — several of which wanted me to speak right away rather than wait for publication of the book! (I foolishly estimated I would be able to knock the book out in three months and have it published within six at the time so I postponed all but one of those speaking engagements.)

Providing a platform for other caregivers to process their anger and frustration and feelings of helplessness really interested me though. I thought, *Wow, maybe I don't actually totally suck for being so honest about how difficult my journey as a caregiver has been! Maybe I can be helpful to other caregivers.*

So, this book, "A Caregiver's Journey" was born and later that summer, the initial steps and outline for The Caregiving Project was launched. It's taken two years instead of six months, but I hope the extra time spent building the platform will prove useful to other caregivers.

I wrote the previous chapter "What To Expect As A Caregiver" with pure, 20/20 hindsight. But I placed it before this section on how to cope with being a caregiver intentionally. Because it's information that I wished I had when I started my caregiving journey more than fifteen years ago.

Putting it first also provides context for some of the coping mechanisms I'm about to suggest.

What I learned what some might call "the hard way" or "on my own" ultimately became the inspiration for this book. Intellectually I knew I wasn't the only one dealing with a parent or loved one with Alzheimer's or some other form of dementia. I was lucky to have an understanding and sympathetic wife, in-laws and even a few friends willing to listen to my trials and tribulations dealing with my mother. But most of our conversations tended to land around various care alternatives, or mutually comforting spiritual platitudes about a similar experience they had with someone they knew.

I realized I'm not alone. Great.

Lots of people have and are going through the exact same thing I am. Great.

So then why am I having so much trouble dealing with it?

The answer is because the mental, emotional and spiritual challenge of watching someone you love deteriorate so completely not only sucks, it's wicked hard, too.

It took me a long time to realize and admit it, but a caregiver's journey with an Alzheimer's and/or dementia patient can be just as difficult as the patient's journey.

But nobody talks about that.

Caregivers typically think they are not "allowed" to talk about themselves. It's natural when taking care of someone else to feel selfish for complaining about it. We don't want to risk being negatively judged by our family and friends so we suppress those feelings.

But that's why every time I finally started talking about my own problems dealing with the challenges, other people immediately opened up and shared their own difficulties dealing with their situations, too.

That's why I decided to write this book specifically for caregivers and why I started my blog — so that other caregivers will have a place to share their story, ask uncomfortable questions, and find community with others dealing with dementia on a day-to-day basis rather than those who are searching for a cure by studying data in a laboratory. Coping with the often very profound and very ugly, very messy effects of someone you love who has the disease is no small task, but to date, there hasn't been a lot of guidance on it.

Caregivers, along with doctors, nurses and friends, naturally tend to think of their patient first. It's easy to find lots of books and advice on:

- How to make them comfortable.

- How to mediate and alleviate the stresses in their lives.

- What drugs, mood stabilizers and anti-psychotic medicine might work.

- How to try to entertain them.

- How to make them happier.

- How to listen to them and calm them down and talk them through their seemingly endless bouts of depression and toxic lashing out.

But I had trouble finding any book that talked about how to do all then and then still find the clarity and the strength to go about my day and accomplish the things that I needed to do.

The fact is, a caregiver, especially a caregiver trying to cope with someone manifesting some of the more toxic behaviours of dementia, absolutely MUST take deliberate and conscious and yes, sometimes even seemingly selfish steps to protect their own mental, spiritual and physical health.

So the first step in how to cope with being a caregiver is to:

Admit to yourself that you are a caregiver. Say it out loud. "My mother (or father, grandmother, or grandfather, spouse, or brother, or sister, or uncle, aunt, or friend) has dementia. They need my help. I am their primary caregiver. It is up to me to either provide or find them the help that they need."

From there it's easier to prepare yourself for what is likely to happen as your loved one's needs increase and process the many unpleasant things you might hear along the way as they do.

Dealing With The Stress Instead of Denying It

I didn't see my stress coming. That afternoon when my phone rang in Flagstaff and I felt a shooting pain in my chest shouldn't have surprised me. But it did. Fortunately, enough to finally do something about it. I didn't know how stressed out I was until I finally started getting short breaks from it last year.

Stress kills.

It does.

It took me a long time to realize it and even longer to admit it, but when I finally did, I absolutely knew it was there.

When it builds up slowly over a long time you don't feel it growing. It simmers like a spiritual fungus just under the surface of your day-to-day life, deep inside your functioning brain.

Fortunately, but also unfortunately, our human bodies and our human brains are designed to cope with whatever environment we find ourselves immersed in.

When the stress in our environment is fast and immediate, like finding the nearest exit when we hear a fire alarm go off, our nervous system shoots into survival mode and stays elevated until whatever threat around us passes or is resolved.

When the stress in our environment is not immediate, but persistent, like holding your hand to a warm radiator and keeping it there as the temperature of the radiator slowly rises, our nervous systems don't warn us when our hand starts to burn.

As I mentioned earlier, the first time I admitted to myself (and to others) that my mother had a problem was Christmas 2004. She called on Christmas Day, after being out with us for a very pleasant Christmas Eve, to abruptly announce that she refused to come over for dinner. She was convinced that I hated her, Laura (my future wife) hated her, and Laura's parents not only hated her but didn't want her there.

There was no rational reason for her to feel that way. No one had said or done a thing. But something inside of her had snapped.

She was so sullen and so vindictive about it that after trying to reason and assure her multiple times that she was mistaken, I gave up and moved on with my life that day. My mother remained sullen and distant for about a week after the incident and brought it up everytime I spoke with her, still convinced of her original accusations. Her brain misfired and created a memory imprint of being mistreated, unwanted and ridiculed and that is what she remembered about that day for years.

As a guy, it didn't make any sense to me when it happened. Or whenever she brought it up. But I couldn't fix it. In her mind I was wrong for hating her AND wrong for arguing with her that I DIDN'T hate her. It was a lose/lose argument that I dealt with by laughing about and simply tried to avoid a repeat of it going forward.

It wasn't the first time my mother had formed a very strong opinion about something that wasn't real. Before that breakdown, Laura and I had both witnessed my mother get piss mad at waiters or waitresses or other strangers for no real reason. Usually it was sort of humorous because it was so surreal. In the months leading up to that Christmas dinner, I heard my mother drop the f-bomb for the first time in my life.

Instead of being concerned, I thought that was rather humorous too.

But finding the humor in my mother's behaviour only worked as a defense mechanism for so long. As the months progressed and the phone conversations started getting longer and more circular, it stopped being funny anymore. All of her friends in her dance class somehow turned on her. But I still found a way to rationalize it. All of her friends in Arlington "betrayed" her somehow. But I still found a way to rationalize, compartmentalize, or ignore that and all of her other bad behavior too. She was getting old. She was 80 … and then she was 81 … and then she was 85 … and then she was 90.

But she was still doing great for 90!

In many ways, by that point, she was doing better than I was. I was becoming 210 pounds of raw nerve and she was still living on her own in a 55+ community. Still cooking, eating right and shopping for her own groceries. Still balancing her checkbooks every month and managing her money. She had become an expert on the city and the senior transit systems in Los Angeles, Arlington and Las Vegas in those ten years. She had moved back and forth across the country two more times pretty much entirely without help. She was still mobile and articulate with the spunk to go to a museum or wherever else she liked entirely on her own. She even flew by herself back East to visit her sister a couple times a year up until she was in her early 90's.

She was doing great. On the outside.

But the dire, despair-filled phone calls had gotten steadily worse. She was constantly furious, or crushed, about something. But I kept trying to fix it. I kept trying to make her happy.

The Problem Is Not The Problem

She'd complain about her TV, I'd buy her a new TV. She'd be briefly elated but then despise me for buying her a TV with a faulty remote just to "torture" her.

I'd show her how to use it again and write down the instructions in a simplified form and then she'd lose them and accuse me of taking them with me, again, just to "torture" her.

When I got tired of listening to her complain about her phone not working (while we were talking on it) I bought her a new phone, one recommended by AARP for older adults. I'd show her how to use it and then re-write the instructions to simplify them. But again, a day or week later I was accused of "torturing" her again.

Obviously, the fact that she moved thirteen (13!) times in twenty-six years wasn't usually because of where she was living. But for me, it was easier to deal with one move at a time because no other solutions were presenting themselves. (She did manage to stay in one place for almost six years until she was evicted)

Where she was living wasn't the problem.

The TV wasn't the problem.

The phone wasn't the problem.

She was just always mad at everything and everyone — especially me, because I was just about the only one who would listen to her for more than ten minutes at that point so I was in her target zone the most. But I didn't know how to deal with it other than to internalize it and try to fix each problem as it came up.

As Mark Twain so aptly said, "Doing the same thing over and over expecting different results is the very definition of insanity."

She refused to admit her age to most people. Everyone said she looked and acted like she was 10-15 years younger than she really was. But, I realize now, although outwardly she seemed to be doing fine, inside, things had radically changed in her brain.

I knew my mother had a problem and for ten years I watched it slowly get worse. I tried to deal with each incident as it came in a loving, caring, problem-solving, rational-as-possible way. I found her great places to live but none of them were ever good enough for very long. Pleasant weekly visits became toilsome. Multiple, desperate, frantic, manically depressed phone calls became routine.

Fourteen years after calling to refuse to come to Christmas dinner in 2004 my blood pressure was spiking and my heart was leaping out of my chest everytime the phone rang.

Stress kills. Which is why it is so important for people dealing with loved ones with Alzheimer's and dementia to keep a close, honest and watchful eye on their own health.

I've had numerous counselors, therapists and eldercare/hospice administrators tell me that 60% of people coping with a parent or loved one's Alzheimer's and dementia end up developing a health condition of their own.

I'm one of them. I've been dealing with my mother's dementia for over 15 years now and that toll started noticeably catching up with me last year.

Although things got progressively worse in the last five years, and most profoundly in the past two, I honestly believe I didn't notice the precipitous decline in my own health because my hand has been on the radiator for over 15 years.

Processing Your Frustration and Finding An Outlet To Scream

During what was intended as a transition period between two jobs I started writing a novel set in the old apartment building where I lived in Venice Beach. The writing flowed. My wife and I were doing okay and she encouraged me to devote myself to my lifelong passion for writing. That novel eventually became my second novel, *FOR RENT: Dangerous Paradise* and was published in 2014.

For me, writing became my therapy. I started a sequel *FOR RENT: Haunted Neon* to my first book and set it in Las Vegas in-between doing a little freelance journalism. I was on the board of directors of a local 501(c)3 literary non-profit by then and about to take the reins as president of the small group. Giving back to my community gave me a sense of purpose above and beyond picking up the phone and coaching my mother out of her latest pit of despair.

After that phone call in Flagstaff that scared me into putting my own mental, physical and spiritual well-being ahead of my mother's, I also drove out into the Mojave Desert and screamed myself hoarse sometimes.

A dead caregiver is the worst caregiver and fortunately I realized that in time to start healing myself before my mother's condition really nosedived off a cliff. I don't know if I would have been able to handle the rest of 2018, or 2019 when she started falling in the middle of the night and the phone would ring cryptically from Paradise, Nevada at 3AM if I wasn't already on the path to wellness.

Forgiving yourself for doing what's best for you when you are caring for someone else is the only way to protect yourself from the guilt and anger and frustration and hopelessness that comes from witnessing a loved one suffering from a degenerative neurological disease that has no cure.

So, again, the first step in how to cope with being a caregiver for someone with dementia (or Alzheimer's) is to:

1. **Admit to yourself that you are a caregiver.** Say it out loud. "My mother (or father, grandmother, or grandfather, spouse, or brother, or sister, or uncle, aunt, or friend) has <dementia>. They need my help. I am their primary caregiver. It is up to me to either provide or find them the help that they need."

The second step is to:

2. **Give yourself permission to be angry**, frustrated, or feel hurt by the things your loved one says to you or accuses you of. Don't bury those hurt feelings or deny that you feel them. Find a way to express that anger before you take it out on someone else around you. Dig below the surface to discover why what they said hurt you. Feel it. Own it. (Scream back at it!!!) Then let it go. Otherwise, it's likely to bubble up and out of you when you least expect it, like at Thanksgiving, or Christmas, or some other time your loved one is standing on your last nerve. Which they will. I guarantee you. Over and over and over again.

Then, you can proceed to the third and most important step which is:

3. **<u>Forgive yourself and admit to others when you need help</u>**. I admit, as a guy, I tried to fix most of my mother's problems more logically than emotionally. Especially in the beginning. Not an entirely terrible problem solving approach, but definitely not the most useful or effective one for a long-term solution either. Getting her into an assisted-living facility, and ultimately into a full-time memory care facility, definitely helped to ease the daily stress of worrying about whether she was safe, getting the proper care that she needed, and had enough to eat. But those facilities came with their own sets of challenges too, so they were not a cure-all for her, or me. But having partners in her care was huge.

Planning For the Future

One of the uglier truths about caring for a loved with Alzheimer's or other type of dementia is **Rule #4 - It's Going To Get Worse Before It Gets Better** (which was presented in Chapter 2).

Unfortunately, this is true for both the patient, and the caregiver.

The first delusional meltdown will lead to more delusional meltdowns and the gaps between future ones will shorten.

One instance of lashing out, hyper-anxiety, or severe paranoia, will eventually become a prevailing personality trait.

Early signs of forgetfulness will likely involve into an inability to form new memories, like using a new TV remote, or new phone, or remembering events or conversations from yesterday.

That forgetfulness will slowly (or sometimes quickly!) trickle back to forgetting events that happened last week, then last month, then last year and degrade all the way to the point of a parent not being able to recognize the face of their own child anymore.

Minor mobility impairments will eventually lead to difficulties walking, the need for a walker, the need for a wheelchair, and ultimately being mostly bedridden.

One bladder control instance will lead to another and another and eventually, usually rather quickly, also involve bowel control problems. Daily diaper changing will become necessary and the risk of UTI's (urinary track infections) will need to be constantly monitored and addressed.

The need to stop by and check-in on your loved one will go from once a week, to twice a week, to daily.

Your loved one will stop remembering to eat and need to have some sort of meal plan where meals are provided.

Trouble eating and swallowing will advance to not be able to eat or swallow.

All of these things sound awful and they are. But the best way to deal with them is to anticipate what your loved one's needs will be in advance so that you, their primary caregiver or legal guardian, can plan and prepare for those transitions.

The BEST FIRST THING a caregiver can do for their loved one is sit down and have a frank and honest discussion about their **end-of-life directives**.

- Do they want to be hooked up to feeding tubes if they can no longer eat?

- Do they want to be put on a ventilator if they start having trouble breathing on their own?

- Do they want to drain their life savings to have pacemakers and kidney replacements and other invasive surgeries?

- How do they feel about right-to-die laws for terminal patients that might exist in the state where they live?

- Do they wish to be cremated, or buried? Large service or small? Or have a destination funeral that is more like a life celebration than a funeral?

If there is any debate within the family about ANY of these wishes, make sure your loved one fills out a formal **Health Care Directive** so that their final wishes are NOT compromised or delayed because of a religious debate between their surviving loved ones when it comes time to make difficult decisions.

The answers to these and other questions like these will provide the caregiver with a vital roadmap for when the ravages of the disease are at their worst.

- If they want a Do Not Resuscitate (DNR) Order in case of a catastrophic event make sure they (or you) get their doctor to fill one out and make multiple copies of it so that they have one on them at all times, you have one, and you have copies to provide the nursing home and assisted-living facilities where they might have to live in the future.

- Make sure they make out a Will and that it is notarized while they are still legally competent. There are multiple free templates available online, but if there are any complicated trusts or other asset holdings it is absolutely worth the expense of hiring an attorney to advise them, and you, through the process.

- Make sure they assign a Power of Attorney for financial and legal affairs BEFORE they can no longer do so for themselves competently.

- Make sure they assign a Power of Healthcare Attorney. This is vitally important and should be someone that they absolutely trust to make decisions in accordance with their Health Care Directive and previously expressed end-of-life wishes. This also helps to avoid one person's religious beliefs, or even an institution's religious beliefs, from interfering in your loved one's final wishes.

- Another excellent thing to have pre-arranged (and pre-paid for) is funeral arrangements. Like with most things in life, the vultures in this world will come out in force to take advantage of a grieving family in their time of need. Having your loved one's funeral arrangements pre-arranged and pre-paid avoids this and also allows for time to shop around and get the best price for the desired arrangements. (Funeral prices vary widely and it is not something that a family needs to argue about or compromise over once the time has come.)

For some people, death is the saddest thing in the world. But, I'm here to tell you that it can also be a blessing. My mother knew what was coming for her. She saw her mother "live" for ten long years as a shell of her former self in a bed, in a nursing home, all alone. She couldn't speak, she couldn't eat or swallow, she didn't recognize anyone, she couldn't breathe on her own, but she was kept alive with machines and tubes until her body finally said enough. My mother dreaded that sort of death for years and made it very plain to me that she never wanted to have to endure what her mother did just for the sake of being alive. My mother, although she grew up a devout Lutheran, believed in reincarnation and actually looked forward to her next spin around our little blue marble in her next life. But no matter what someone's spiritual beliefs are, making sure that when their time comes their passing to the other side is as quick and painless as possible is something I think anyone who has watched someone die would say.

For me, after my mother died the end of April 2020 during the early stage of the Covid-19 pandemic (for the record, she didn't die from Covid, Alzheimer's was the main cause listed on her death certificate), the opportunity to begin remembering her for who she really was, how she lived and kicked ass in this life, was reborn. Was I sad? Certainly. But dementia and Alzheimer's are uniquely cruel diseases. In many ways I had lost her ten, even fifteen years before she actually died one month shy of her 97th birthday. So the opportunity to start remembering her again for who she was has been a blessing in the months since she passed.

The fact that our digital picture frame in the living room, which has at least 50 different pictures on it of places my wife and I have been, keeps sticking on the one of my mother laughing joyously with her sister at our wedding just confirms that in many ways, she is more alive to me today than she was last year.

I hope this provides some comfort to those still on their caregiving journey now. It will get worse before it gets better. But then you'll find the right place for your loved one. They will get the care that they need. The stress, yours and theirs, will melt away if and when you let it.

CHAPTER 6

CARE FACILITIES AND TREATMENT OPTIONS

As I mentioned earlier, I am not a doctor, or nurse, nor have I ever worked at an eldercare facility. I have certainly spent a lot of time inside quite a few though! Both as someone checking up one one of their residents and as a featured author. As discussed in CHAPTER 3, I have not presented the definitions of dementia and Alzheimer's from a clinical or medical point of view either. But rather from someone who has seen a difference between what those two words have meant to me and most other people I've spoken with outside of the medical and eldercare professions.

When speaking with doctors and nurses, and even administrators or other staff at eldercare facilities, it is important to be as precise with our language as possible in order to help our loved one get the best care possible. I can't tell you how many times I was personally thanked and appreciated for being open and honest about the personality and behavior traits that my mother was exhibiting. Especially the less pleasant ones!

That in turn helped them be honest with me about what they observed.

Which in turn helped determine the best course of action and meds for her.

Describing symptoms, rather than just labeling them, is extremely important when it comes to prescription meds.

I avoided saying that my mother had Alzheimer's because for a long time she wasn't exhibiting the usual characteristic of Alzheimer's — forgetfulness. This became increasingly important because as I found out, often the hard way, not all antipsychotic medicines are the same. Many can in fact work against one each other. Or worse, in conflict with other medications.

Because of our aging population, Alzheimer's and dementia research is blazing forward at an amazing rate and in dozens of different directions right now. There are several promising looking therapies on the horizon and some promising looking preventive care measures currently being introduced and studied and tested.

New terminology for different aspects of the disease is being introduced all the time. As a caregiver advances through the stages of the disease with their loved one, whether they are providing *formal care* or *informal care*, or trying to determine whether their loved one needs *assisted living* or *memory care*, understanding some of the nuances of the terminology is important so that meetings with doctors and nurses and other caregivers can be more productive.

Since 2015, researchers have been able to image the entire disease process of dementia like Alzheimer's from the start of the tangles (the tau proteins that collapse and twist) and the lumps of amyloid proteins that build up in the space between nerve cells within the neural network of the human brain. Hopefully one day this advanced imaging technology may unlock a way to slow or even reverse these proteins and plaques from forming.

But that day has not arrived yet.

So, to better understand the different types of services that different care facilities offer, it's important for the primary caregiver or legal guardian of a dementia patient to first understand some of the present-day treatment options for patients suffering from Alzheimer's (or other type of dementia) in order to make an informed decision about what's best for their loved one <u>and</u> themselves as well.

Treatment Options

As a son who wanted his mother to stay as healthy and happy and active as possible in her later years, I took the advice of many doctors about prescription medications for my mother's debilitating mood swings, paranoia, anxiety, anger and episodic rage. I am not going to list all the ones that we tried, but let's just say that it was several of the most popular ones on the market and none of them, not one, worked for her.

The common side effect for most mood stabilizing and anti-anxiety medications that are on the market today is depression.

For someone who was already suffering from delusional thoughts about how everyone around her was conspiring against her, and also periodically slipping into a deep, deep well of despair, "medicine" that just made her profound bouts of depression worse proved, for her at least, NOT to be the answer.

What worked far better for my mother, and from what I've seen from being an author invited into dozens of retirement facilities to talk about and discuss my other books, is active, daily engagement. Growing old sucks. A person's sense of self-worth can deteriorate and disappear without the demands of a job, raising children or helping others create something in this world.

When the reasons for living become blurry and ill-defined, it's important to keep an older person active, or interested in new things. Although many people with the genetic tendency for Alzheimer's begin to exhibit early signs of the disease, like forgetfulness, in their mid-60's, my mother's forgetfulness didn't become pronounced until she was in her early 90's. **Almost every single one of her doctors said that the relatively late onset of her dementia was directly attributable to her years of dancing**, especially later in her life AFTER she turned 60. Because dancing, especially step-specific dancing like a waltz or rumba or line dancing, as opposed to free-style, requires the brain and the body to coordinate. For the step to be remembered and executed in a correct sequence while listening and timing each step to the beat of the music.

The other thing that worked heavily in my mother's favor, her doctors said and I concur with because I saw it with my own eyes to be true, **was my mother's adherence to a heart healthy diet** high in omega-3 fatty acids, vitamin C (she drank a glass of fresh, premium orange juice everyday up until she was at least 94) and leafy green vegetables.

Did the fatty acids from all the fish she ate, along with the citric acids of all the orange juice she drank, help burn away the sticky plaques trying to form in her brain? Maybe. But it makes sense. Citric acid is used to kill bacteria and clean corroded metal so it's not impossible to make a connection that it might be beneficial for keeping the fragile neural pathways of the human brain clear and clean.

The other factor several of her doctors mentioned, and I corroborated in the research that I've done, **was my mother's lifelong interest in music, specifically classical music.**

Studies have shown that puzzle games like crosswords, sudoku, along with reading and listening to complex musical patterns is a great mental work out for both older and younger brains too. My mother was an avid reader of the newspaper her whole life. After her retirement she had the time to add books to her daily reading. She started having trouble remembering what she had just read around the time she turned 90, but she kept reading the paper everyday up until she was 94 and didn't entirely give up on books until she was 95.

It took me a long time to realize that a glass of wine and a new book was the best therapy for my mother.

Yes, while at the height of the toxicity of her dementia when she was 94 and 95, a strong anti-anxiety pill could calm her down by basically knocking her out, that pill or any others like it was not the best solution on a daily basis.

Studies have also shown that the human brain is stimulated by reminders of the past (sights, sounds, smells, etc.) and that the electrical activity in our brains actually increases when an old memory is stimulated or accessed.

Music is one of the easiest non-invasive tools to make a dementia patient's life more enjoyable.

I found music to be a particularly great stimulus tool (and pacifier) with my mother because when she was in the middle stage of her disease and at her most toxic, it was difficult to want to be around her. But my wife and I found that we could take her to concerts by the Henderson Symphony Orchestra at the (now gone) Pavilion in Green Valley Ranch here in Las Vegas to listen to the classical music that she was drawn to her whole life and that compelled her to become an usher at the Kennedy Center after she retired. Those pleasant evenings stirred pleasant memories for my mother and rarely ever triggered her to lash out at me or anyone else.

Sadly, when she was in the later stages of her disease, she didn't remember ever being an usher at the Kennedy Center. Classical music didn't stir the same fond memories for her that it once did. But, after a lifetime of saying that she "didn't get" jazz and didn't like it, she became a fan of jazz. So much so that she would even dance and bob a little in the car, and even later, in her wheelchair, whenever I played it for her. (I discovered this by happy accident because the station I listen to most in my car is a jazz station and it usually comes on when I start the engine.)

In doing research for this book, I found that some of those same studies I just mentioned also discovered that the human brain, no matter how old or damaged, actually builds new neural pathways when exposed to new stimuli.

So even if your loved one previously loved one type of music but hated another, keeping music in your caregiving toolbox throughout your journey can prove very beneficial for them and as well as you the caregiver. (So go ahead and play your favorite music that your loved one used to hate!) Playing the music they always loved while they still remember that they love it can improve quality time with them. Then, when they've slipped beyond remembering what they once liked and didn't like, playing the music they might have always said they never cared for can actually boost their mood and actually stimulate their brain and make them feel happy.

Of course, many older people develop hearing problems so music is not a universal solution.

In that case, my advice would be to try a favorite color for a scarf or item of clothing to serve the same purpose. When the favorite colored scarf doesn't work anymore, try a different color, especially a color they never claimed to like before.

Another substitute for music is to activate their brains by experimenting with different smells. My mother always loved the fragrance of roses. But in her later years she expressed more fondness towards lavender.

Different tastes might be another good sensory experiment. Although most Alzheimer's patients develop severe difficulty with swallowing so experimenting with different tastes probably wouldn't work with late stage Alzheimer's patients.

Staying up-to-date with the latest therapies and treatment options for Alzheimer's and other dementia is an exciting and hopeful, ever changing landscape because it's a constantly evolving area of research. Fortunately, more and more resources are coming online every month to help understand a disease that is affecting millions and millions more people every year.

Care Facilities

When it comes to in-home care options, assisted living, or memory-care facilities (remember there's a difference), treatment strategies and medications, it's important for the caregiver to ALWAYS keep in mind that healthcare, as it currently is in the United States in 2021, is driven by profit, not caring.

It's also important to keep in mind that most healthcare workers are NOT paid well. (This is why your loved one's valuables are at risk of going missing in care facilities.) But, the company or agency or facility they work for is typically paid exceptionally well—often through a combination of government grants, your loved one's insurance, on top of the additional charges that you or your loved one pays to them directly.

As tempting as it sometimes is, it's important not to take out your frustrations or anger on the healthcare workers taking care of your loved one. They are doing their best under difficult, demanding, often no-win situations for barely more than minimum wage. So just be aware that any advice you might get from them is in the company's best interest, not yours or your loved one's.

Since Medicare and many private/company health insurers only pay for short-stay care (typically anywhere from 30-100 days) many people are forced to become poor (burn through all their assets) in order to qualify for Medicaid. Medicaid pays for long-term nursing home care but not emergency surgeries and prevention services covered by Medicare. Being forced to choose between Medicare coverage and Medicaid coverage is not an easy choice to make and it's one that often leads well-meaning caregivers to feeling forced into caring for their loved one in their own home.

Choosing to care for an aging person that may have other health issues besides just Alzheimer's is a huge, life-changing decision that should not be made because of some misguided attempt "to do what's best for them." Such a choice will not only fundamentally and radically change your home environment, it is guaranteed to add an unimaginable amount of stress to it as well—for you and the loved ones that you live with. For one thing, changing diapers for an adult is not the same as changing diapers on an infant. Making sure that your full-time, in-home patient is fed and cleaned and entertained on top of making sure they aren't falling down or choking on something will disrupt your life more than you can probably handle. That's why it's vitally important to know what your loved one's wishes are BEFORE that crossroads is faced. **(See Chapter 5 - How To Cope - Planning For the Future)**.

Having an Advanced Directive, or DNR (Do Not Resuscitate), and knowing what your loved ones feelings and preferences are about having things like feeding tubes, pacemakers, oxygen ventilators, and other ugly, painful medical devices attached to them just to keep them alive, will make the decisions a primary caregiver or legal guardian has to face so, so much easier. Plus, most parents never want to be a burden on their children. Making a decision that puts them in that position will nine times out of ten cause even more resentment and depression on their part.

Even though the conversation(s) to determine what your loved one's end-of-life wishes are won't be easy, if you avoid having them I guarantee you will regret it.

Trying to get a surviving spouse, brother, sister, or your own siblings to all agree on the same fate for a loved one dying from the effects of Alzheimer's is not a battlefield anyone will come off of unscathed.

My advice is to always seek professional care for your loved one outside of your own home if at all possible. A caregiver's home is often their last and only sanctuary. Jeopardizing that sanctuary violates Rule #1 of being a caregiver. Because if you don't look out for your own health and well-being, no one else will.

You might be told that a memory care facility requires an official diagnosis of Alzheimer's, or other dementia, from a doctor to be admitted. Some doctors are quick to diagnose Alzheimer's. Others are hesitant and help you understand the ramifications of doing so.

Watch out for doctors who are quick to diagnose Alzheimer's.

An official diagnosis of Alzheimer's (or other dementia like Lewy Body or Mixed Dementia) means that your loved one is being declared legally incompetent. It is a diagnosis that is virtually impossible to have reversed because no other doctor is going to put his or her reputation and medical license on the line to do so.

In most states, being declared incompetent legally escalates the type of care that is required for that person. Typically that escalation comes with a significant increase in costs. Many 55+ senior communities have costs that are roughly in line with your local housing rental market. Ones that provide extra services like activity directors and bus trips generally run anywhere from 20-50% higher than the local housing rental market. Assisted-living facilities that provide meals, on staff nurses, bathing and grooming assistance, along with other services and activities are typically about double that of the 55+ communities. Full-time memory care facilities typically cost double, or even triple! what the assisted-living facilities cost. So being diagnosed as incompetent due to Alzheimer's or other dementia can mean a big, <u>BIG</u> increase in costs for care.

The important thing for caregivers to remember about treatments, medications and care facilities for a patient suffering from any form of dementia is that it is a growing business not only in the United States, but also around the world. But, believe it or not, that's actually a good thing. Because since it is a growing business and more and more research is being directed towards it, that means there is not only more competition for your caregiving dollars, there is also hope.

There are many excellent facilities and services out there already and they are dramatically expanding in every single country around the world. But it is also a minefield of competing interests and information. Finding the treatment and care that works best for you and your loved one requires research, persistence and finding a support network that knows and understands your unique set of challenges.

The best treatment is the one that works the best for you. And the best care facility is the one where your loved one is happiest and the most safe from themselves and others.

Hopefully though, now you have more tools to find each of those things than you did before you picked up my book!

CHAPTER 7

MAKING THE MOST OUT OF THE TIME THAT'S LEFT

The baseline prognosis many doctors currently give for people diagnosed with Alzheimer's is 3 to 9 years. But different studies have shown that is only a statistical estimate based on a history of limited and incomplete data.

Many people live with the disease much longer.

Other people deteriorate much faster.

As in my mother's case, some dementias can begin to exhibit years before the forgetfulness of Alzheimer's does. My journey dealing with her increasingly anxiety-driven behaviour, as the degenerative neurological decay progressed in her brain, lasted over 15 years. Taking into account the fact that she moved back and forth across the country five times in eight years, it was probably more like 20 years.

The demands of her journey evolved slowly but steadily. Her toxicity increased ahead of any decline in her capabilities. But then a new set of demands presented themselves once the toxicity subsided and the forgetfulness and physical decay of Alzheimer's began attacking the parts of the brain that control motor skills and bodily functions.

It wasn't easy. My caregiving journey had to adapt to those transitions and changes too.

Looking back at my experience, I'm glad that I didn't let my mother's toxicity completely ruin our relationship. As the number of her "good days" became less and fewer, I still planned events and outings with her. Even during the years when she was the fiercest about keeping her independence, I did my best to respect that and still surround her in a cocoon of support.

I knew she had it in her to have fun and fortunately my wife knew it too and focused on creating new good memories for us. Laura thought of specific things my mother would (or at least might) enjoy, she pitched them to me and then either she or I would pitch them to my mother.

We often let my mother choose in order to empower her and give her a sense of control in her otherwise crumbling world.

By the time my mother finally admitted that she was slipping, she was already pretty far gone. For years she denied it and blamed others for everything that was changing in her life. All that denial and blame destroyed her relationship with her sister, all her friends in D.C., Virginia, California and Nevada, and strained our relationship beyond measure too.

However, despite all the terrible phone calls and arguments and all the parties and holidays that she spitefully sabotaged, we still managed to have some good times.

Making the most of the quality time that's left with a loved one suffering from Alzheimer's or other type of dementia is important because:

- I didn't know that the last time we had my mother over to our house that it was going to be the last time.

- I didn't know that the last time we took our puppy Reno over to visit her (and the other residents) at her last memory care facility that it was going to be the last time.

- And I didn't know that the last time we took her out to lunch and were able to enjoy a beer together that it was going to be the last time.

But they were and now when I recall those memories, I remember just about every detail about each and every one of those times and others.

In some diseases, like cancer or diabetes or kidney failure, a prognosis for the amount of quality time someone has left is often pretty accurate. It's horrible and gut-wrenching but plans to see family and friends one last time, even plans for a dignified end, can be set. Unfortunately, the same is NOT true with Alzheimer's.

Once someone has been diagnosed with Alzheimer's, whether it's informally because the disease hasn't progressed to the Late Stage yet, or formally because it has and your loved one has started falling down, their speech has become unintelligible, and they've started having trouble swallowing or breathing on their own, their time on this little blue marble of ours is nearing its end even if you decide to hook them up to ventilators and feeding tubes to prolong their misery.

Due to advances in our medical expertise, someone can survive on feeding tubes and oxygen infusions and be bedridden for years. My grandmother lived to be 101. She was bedridden, couldn't eat and could barely speak for the last eleven years of her life. Even as a young boy, I could tell by looking in her gray blue eyes she was dying to die.

That is not what I am calling quality of life.

Quality of life has different meanings for different people though.

Does quality of life mean alive but living with constant pain?

Does quality of life mean living with modest, or relatively little pain?

Does quality of life mean being able to walk around?

Being able to use the bathroom?

Being able to live at home?

Being able to recognize friends and family?

Being able to participate in social gatherings?

Personally, a good quality of life definition for me means being: pain free without being sedated; able to walk with minimal assistance; keep up with personal hygiene; recognize friends and family; and able to participate in social gatherings.

My mother was able to do most of those things up until about the last year of her life. The fact that she started telling everyone who would listen that she wanted to die long, long before that probably had more to do with her own personal cosmology than the mixed dementia. She had an amazing life. When she noticed she was starting to slip, she fought it, she denied it, she resisted the changes that needed to happen to keep her safe and comfortable, but she was ready and longing to go.

I remember the last time my wife and I took her on a picnic to our favorite spot near the Valley of Fire in the Lake Mead Recreation Area. It was a place that my mother dearly loved and often told people about. When it started getting close to sunset I remarked that it looked like it might be a fantastic, very colorful one. And my mother said, "So what? I've seen all the sunsets I ever want to see."

She had an amazing knack for being poetically morbid sometimes. Did she ruin the moment? Yes. But the poignancy of the remark made me both sad and at the same time, helped me understand her better.

I know whenever I decide that I've seen enough sunsets, it will be my time to go too.

We drove back home and stopped for ice cream at our favorite place in the little town of Overton. I didn't know at the time it was going to be our last picnic together, but I suggested we stop. Of course, my mother didn't want to. Which was just her being contrary because she knew we knew that she loved ice cream. She wasn't dealing with any weight related issues, so it was an indulgence she often allowed herself. I used her own psychology on her. "This might be the last time you'll have a chance to have Blue Bell ice cream. Remember how good it was the last time?"

Whether she actually did remember or not, I will never know. But she said she did (I was pulling into the parking lot anyways because I wanted some) so I gave her two choices. She could sit in the car while Laura and I went in or come in and get some "free" ice cream because I was paying. Laura of course offered to stay in the car with my mother to be nice, which sort of blew up my goal, but even my grumpy-bump mother who had just announced she had seen enough beautiful sunsets in her life couldn't resist the idea of free ice cream.

Even the ravages of dementia couldn't make rain clouds out of that choice and it was literally like taking a kid into a candy store.

Except the kid was my suddenly elated 94-year-old mother who must have tried at least five flavors before picking one.

Making the most of whatever time is left is a personal choice. But it is a choice that carries along with a finite time limit.

Although towards the end, my relationship with my mother involved constantly mending the new fences that arose (almost daily) rather than old ones, I'm glad I learned by then to stay focused on the present rather than the past. In many situations, a parent or other loved one's slide into Alzheimer's or other type of dementia is an opportunity to mend old long-standing disagreements, slights and feuds within the family. But sometimes it isn't. Sometimes those repairs don't come until after the journey is over.

Families get torn apart and sides get taken for countless reasons. When communication suffers, the anger and separation felt between all the players often lingers and lasts far beyond reason and becomes a habit, not necessarily a desire.

When the good, or not so good, dynamics of a family or group of close friends get disrupted because of a leading figure within the family or group having health issues, communication is forced. Problem resolution requires talking, talking requires listening, listening leads to understanding and understanding often leads to forgiveness. Forgiveness makes compromises easier to make, especially when they need to be made for the good of the person in their decline.

The associated challenges the primary caregiver(s) face have to be dealt with too. But as long as the old stuff is not allowed to sour progress, eventually a new attitude of cooperation and/or mutual need can develop. Sometimes even to the point where the old stuff, or at least some of the old stuff is forgiven and a new start is agreed to.

Families that get pulled back together to care for, or mourn, a loved one, hopefully always, eventually, rejoice in the life that touched them all. In our modern, media driven, news-byte world that reconnection opportunity can easily be lost. So it is important to be mindful of making the most of the time that is left.

Good Things To Do Before It's Too Late

- Encourage visits and phone calls with long lost family members.

- Plan, arrange and host story telling visits over coffee or other favorite beverage.

- Ask what they feel like doing and keep a list.

- Do as many of those things as possible no matter how inconvenient.

- Take pictures, record video of them telling favorite family stories, hold their hand.

I didn't start thinking of good things to do until it was almost too late. It's something I wish I had been more aware of. But, looking back, I don't have too many regrets. I'll always remember driving my mother across the country when she moved from Maryland to southern California and talking the whole way. I took her to Sweden one last time and to the Hermitage Museum in St. Petersburg while she could still enjoy it. She dressed up as a pirate for my pirate-themed wedding in Las Vegas. She watched our golden retriever grow from a puppy into the warmest, best pillow of fur in the world. After she moved to Las Vegas, we enjoyed concerts and shows, buffets and jackpots, and exploring art and historical museums here together.

Along the way, I hung in there. I listened to her rant and rave, I did my best to fix all her real and imagined problems. But in-between all that there were a lot of laughs and we had many, many shared good times.

Towards the end, after I finally began to understand and deal with the emotional, psychological, medical and financial demands of being a caregiver, I was able to distance and gain a little perspective. As previously discussed in **CHAPTER 4 - What To Expect**

As A Caregiver, the final two stages of Alzheimer's are not easy and not pretty.

In my mother's case, as with many who suffer from Alzheimer's and other dementias, the dramatic decline in the end preceded her actual passing by less than two years. That was a long, agonizing period of constant, escalating uncertainty while we were living it, but looking back now, it went by relatively quickly.

I wish I had the presence of mind to start writing down the old family stories that my mother liked to tell. Stories from her days living on the farm, from her wild and crazy single days in Washington, D.C. in the 1950's, to her perspective on things like music, and the advent of TV, the Sixties, the Viet Nam War, and things that I was part of like our annual summer vacations to the beach, and helping me with my paper routes, and driving me off to college, and visiting me when I lived in Manhattan.

During the process of writing this book, I've discovered how much I didn't know about caring for someone with dementia.

Looking back on my experience has helped me figure out:

- What I wish I had known from the beginning,

- How much I found out late and too late,

- and how I can help other caregivers

Writing this book is, in a significant way, my memorial to my mother. Even though it's written from my perspective about what I learned about Alzheimer's, dementia and being a caregiver, it has provided a framework in which to chronicle and give tribute to at least some of my mother's amazing, mostly happy, very, <u>very</u> courageous life.

I'm fortunate in being able to do that since I have been a writer, videographer and amateur historian for many, many years.

To conclude this section on Making The Most of the Time That Is Left, my best advice is to plan as many concerts, picnics, ice creams, holidays, family get-togethers, and libations as you can with your loved one because you <u>will not</u> know which time turns out to be the last time you had the opportunity to do these kinds of things — until after it's too late.

I firmly believe that one of the best gifts we can give to ourselves as caregivers is to make as many new, good memories as possible, as soon as possible, so that they can be treasured years from now after the harder, more unpleasant memories have faded.

Although the primary gift we need to give our patient, our extended family and especially ourselves remains: Take care of yourself and plan for the future! Don't be a dead caregiver! Be a great caregiver!

AFTERWORD

Thank you for reading my book. My mother's long struggle with dementia and Alzheimer's was incredibly challenging and stressful for both her, the patient, and me, her son and primary caregiver. I've found it very therapeutic to share my journey as a caregiver and I hope that in some way my hard lessons learned will be of help to other caregivers. I've found that when I share my story, people come forward eager to share theirs, to let it bubble up to the surface and say the things they need to say. That's good therapy for all of us in my humble opinion so I always welcome and encourage it because I learned, from not dealing with my stress, that we need to process it not bury it.

If you would like to share or talk about your journey, your successes or your challenges, I invite you to visit my blog, **The Caregiving Project** (www.thecaregivingproject.com). I hope it can become a caregiving community and resource center to stay up-to-date on news related to eldercare, planning strategies, stress management tips, and help to find other information specifically geared towards caring for the caregivers of dementia and Alzheimer's patients.

GLOSSARY OF TERMS

Alzheimer's Disease (AD) — Alzheimer's Disease was first identified as "pre-senile dementia" over one hundred years ago by a German psychiatrist and surgeon named Alois Alzheimer. In 1901 he had a patient named Auguste Deter who, because of her behavioral problems, was a permanent resident of a mental asylum in Frankfurt, Germany. He observed her for five years, and when she died in April of 1906 he dissected her brain along with two other surgeons and discovered evidence of hard, microscopic plaques and platelets in the areas of her brain that control cognitive and bodily function. Although Alzheimer's has become synonymous with forgetfulness in practical use, other symptoms, such as hyper-anxiety, paranoia, and rage can and usually do present in later stages.

Dementia — is not a specific type of disease (like Alzheimer's), but rather a group of different diseases associated with neurological decay that cause lapses in reasoning, memory, behaviour and body function. In practical use it often is used to refer to symptoms other than forgetfulness.

———————

Formal Care — formal care involves medical professionals, either via the services of a facility that provides a day-to-day level of caregiving with other medical partners, or via hospice care arrangements where care professionals visit the home where the patient is living.

Informal Care — informal care generally involves someone without formal training who provides support, or periodic support, to an elderly person or family member. This kind of care can also come from friends and local community organizations, but most often it's primarily spouses, followed by adult children and other relatives.

———————

Fifty-five (55) Plus — refers to housing communities, either apartments or houses, where at least one resident must be 55 years of age or older to qualify to live there. Residents must be able to live on their own independently, with limited assistance. Typically, 55-Plus communities have one or several different community centers, rooms and an Activities Program that includes various exercise options, excursions, games and entertainment. Some offer prepared meals, some don't. Some offer limited nursing advice or check-ins, but most typically do not. Thus, they are much cheaper than assisted-living or memory-care facilities.

Assisted-Living Facility — an assisted-living facility is generally a retirement home for senior citizens where one all-inclusive price covers their room, utilities, meals and activities, with tiered services for those who need a daily nurse or nurse practitioner to help with their medical equipment, personal hygiene, feeding themselves, keeping up with their medications (if any), walking, or other challenges. Generally residents are free to have a car and come and go as they please as long as they agree to check out and check back in whenever they go anywhere. Weekly, or at least bi-weekly doctor visits are also a common service that is offered as are regular updates to a primary caregiver or legal guardian.

Memory Care Facility — a memory care facility covers all the services of an assisted-living facility except that it has locks on all the outer doors so that they cannot leave the facility unescorted. Patients are regularly checked on by a nurse or nurse practitioner if they are bedridden or choose to stay in their own room rather than gather in the group room with the other residents.

Hospice — hospice can either be an in-home service where a nurse or nurse practitioner visits the private home where the dementia patient is living for a certain number of hours per day, or an extensive level of care within a facility for a bedridden or dying patient within an assisted-living or memory care facility.

ACKNOWLEDGMENTS

I would like to thank fellow authors Stephen Murray and Nancy Nelson for encouraging me to set aside other projects and write this book. Although it was harder than I expected, in the end, writing it helped me put some perspective on what it meant to be a caregiver and it helped me process the changes in my mother's personality that I had to contend with, so for that gift of healing I thank you both.

I also want to thank all of those who encouraged me to keep working on this book whenever I thought what I had to say wasn't important because I wasn't a doctor or nurse. For that I would like to especially thank my beautiful wife Laura, and fellow fiction and non-fiction author Paul Papa, and my other friends and colleagues at Writers of Southern Nevada who helped me find my voice on this project.

Lastly, I would like to thank all the activity directors and nursing staff at the facilities where my mother lived for being so compassionate and understanding in their caregiving roles. Their encouragement and kind words inspired me to share my journey in the hope that it might help other caregivers on theirs.

ABOUT THE AUTHOR

Eric James Miller was born in Washington, D.C., grew up in Bethesda, Maryland and has lived in St. Paul, Berlin, New York, Denver, Los Feliz and Venice Beach in L.A.. He currently calls the neon corridors of Las Vegas home but is open to suggestions. His other books include the paranormal murder mystery *For Rent: Dangerous Paradise* and the road trip comedy *The Metaphysics of Nudity*.

Visit his author website (www.ericjamesmiller.com) for more information about his other work, or visit his blog (www.thecaregivingproject.com) where he covers topics related to caregiving for loved ones with dementia or Alzheimer's and lists upcoming talks and presentations on caring for caregivers.